FAST FACTS ABOUT
THE GYNECOLOGIC EXAM
FOR NURSE PRACTITIONERS

R. "Mimi" Clarke Secor, MS, MEd, RN, FNP-C, FAANP, is a family nurse practitioner specializing in women's health at Newton Wellesley ObGyn, Newton, Massachusetts, and is a visiting scholar at the William F. Connell School of Nursing at Boston College. She is a national speaker and consultant to advanced practice clinicians, president emerita and senior advisor for Nurse Practitioner Associates of Continuing Education (NPACE), and a national radio host on ReachMD. Her 35 years of clinical experience have included emergency care, college health, private practice, prison nursing, and rural clinic nursing. Before working for 7 years at Bethel Family Clinic, in Bethel, Alaska, she operated an independent Boston-area nurse practitioner practice for 12 years. Ms. Secor has extensive media experience, has won several awards, has published numerous articles and book chapters, and is co-author of *Advanced Health Assessment of Women: Clinical Skills and Procedures, 2nd edition* (2010, Springer Publishing Company).

Heidi Collins Fantasia, PhD, RN, WHNP-BC, is an assistant professor in the School of Health and Environment, Department of Nursing at the University of Massachusetts, Lowell, and a visiting scholar at the William F. Connell School of Nursing at Boston College. Dr. Fantasia is a women's health nurse practitioner who provides contraceptive and reproductive health care for a Title X family planning clinic in northeastern Massachusetts. She has over 20 years of clinical nursing experience, including inpatient obstetrics and advanced practice women's health care in both private and public health settings. Dr. Fantasia has published and presented nationally and internationally on a variety of topics related to women's health and conducts research in the area of reproductive health.

FAST FACTS ABOUT THE GYNECOLOGIC EXAM FOR NURSE PRACTITIONERS

Conducting the GYN Exam in a Nutshell

R. "Mimi" Clarke Secor, MS, MEd, RN, FNP-C, FAANP

Heidi Collins Fantasia, PhD, RN, WHNP-BC

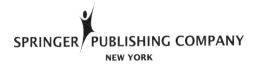

SPRINGER PUBLISHING COMPANY
NEW YORK

Springer Publishing Company, LLC
11 West 42nd Street
New York, NY 10036
www.springerpub.com

Acquisitions Editor: Margaret Zuccarini
Composition: S4Carlisle Publishing Services

ISBN: 978-0-8261-0780-0
E-book ISBN: 978-0-8261-0781-7

12 13 14/ 5 4 3 2 1

The author and the publisher of this work have made every effort to use sources believed to be reliable to provide information that is accurate and compatible with the standards generally accepted at the time of publication. Because medical science is continually advancing, our knowledge base continues to expand. Therefore, as new information becomes available, changes in procedures become necessary. We recommend that the reader always consult current research and specific institutional policies before performing any clinical procedure. The author and publisher shall not be liable for any special, consequential, or exemplary damages resulting, in whole or in part, from the readers' use of, or reliance on, the information contained in this book. The publisher has no responsibility for the persistence or accuracy of URLs for external or third-party Internet Web sites referred to in this publication and does not guarantee that any content on such Web sites is, or will remain, accurate or appropriate.

Library of Congress Cataloging-in-Publication Data

Secor, Mimi Clarke.
  Fast facts about the gynecologic exam for nurse practitioners : conducting the GYN exam in a nutshell / R. "Mimi" Clarke Secor, Heidi Collins Fantasia.
    p. ; cm.
  Includes bibliographical references.
  ISBN 978-0-8261-0780-0—ISBN 0-8261-0780-X—ISBN 978-0-8261-0781-7 (e-book)
  I. Fantasia, Heidi Collins. II. Title.
    [DNLM: 1. Gynecological Examination—nursing—Handbooks. 2. Nurse
    Practitioners—Handbooks. WP 39]
  618.1'0231—dc23

                                                                          2012010065

Special discounts on bulk quantities of our books are available to corporations, professional associations, pharmaceutical companies, health care organizations, and other qualifying groups. If you are interested in a custom book, including chapters from more than one of our titles, we can provide that service as well.

For details, please contact:
Special Sales Department, Springer Publishing Company, LLC
11 West 42nd Street, 15th Floor, New York, NY 10036-8002
Phone: 877-687-7476 or 212-431-4370; Fax: 212-941-7842
Email: sales@springerpub.com

Printed in the United States of America by Hamilton Printing

Contents

Part III: In-Office Diagnostic Testing

Appendices

Foreword

This is an extraordinarily down to earth and useful guide for both novice clinicians and experienced clinicians who are presented with challenging patient situations. The format facilitates both a rapid review immediately prior to stepping into the examination room, as well as a more leisurely study in anticipation of a new clinical challenge or a prospective roster of patients.

The authors have both synthesized and explicated the most important aspects of preparation for, and conduction of, a gynecologic examination under what are sometimes less than ideal circumstances. Their writing is succinct, clear, and easy to read and meets their goal of providing guidance for novice clinicians, as well as providing a quick review for experienced clinicians about to examine patients with unusual or unfamiliar characteristics.

Most of all, this book is a gold mine for clinicians committed to delivering the best possible care to women who present with a wide range of characteristics and challenges. Equally so, it should become a must-have book for novice clinicians as they struggle to make it through their first solo gynecologic examination, and move on to mastering the art of caregiving

as well as the science of providing the best possible individualized care for each woman across the life span.

Joellen W. Hawkins, RN, WHNP-BC, PhD
Professor Emeritus, Boston College,
William F. Connell School of Nursing
Writer-in-Residence, Simmons College School of Nursing
and Health Sciences

Preface

Many advanced practice clinicians (NPs, PAs, CNMs) lack confidence in their women's health skills and may be particularly apprehensive and unsure of their gynecologic exam skills. We've written this book because there is a great need for more practical information about how to improve the advanced practice clinician's gynecologic exam skills.

Fast Facts About the Gynecologic Exam for Nurse Practitioners represents the coauthors' more than four decades of combined clinical experience in women's health and teaching nurse practitioners and other advanced practice clinicians how to perform gynecologic examinations.

This practical guide is designed in an "easy-to-follow" format well suited for the busy clinician looking to refine his or her skills, or for students just learning how to perform a gynecologic exam and their instructors/preceptors who are assisting them.

This book is divided into chapters that each contain key learning objectives and content related to the specific aspect of the gynecologic exam being discussed.

We have included detailed suggestions, approaches, and step-by-step sequences on how to perform the various aspects of the gynecologic exam. Tapping into our vast combined clinical experiences, we've included many practical suggestions both in the body of the text and in the "Fast Facts in a Nutshell" sections of each chapter. These special "Fast Facts" sections contain clinical pearls intended to help clinicians improve their skills so they can conduct a better exam. There are also helpful figures to illustrate information and procedures being discussed.

The text and appendices provide valuable guidelines and documents, including suggestions and strategies for various gynecologic exam challenges and dealing with special populations, a vaginal microscopy flow sheet and summary of how to perform this test and document your results, the new cervical cancer screening guidelines, how to perform an anal Pap smear, and patient education guidelines for vulvovaginal self-care.

This book will help advanced practice clinicians develop and refine their gynecologic examination skills so they can perform a more accurate, patient-centered exam with confidence. This will be a welcome resource, especially for students and their instructors.

Acknowledgments

Thanks to my coauthor, Dr. Heidi Fantasia, who is a great writer and with whom it was a pleasure to work on this project. I am indebted to my patients I've encountered over the years. They are a source of inspiration as I continually learn so much from them. Thank you to my friends, students, and nurse practitioner colleagues for their insight, inspiration, support, and friendship. Special thanks to Dr. Joellen Hawkins and Carine Luxama, NP, for help in editing the manuscript, especially during the final weeks. Finally, thanks to my family, including my husband Mike, daughter Katherine, and mother Irene Clarke, for their unconditional love and for sharing me with my work.

R. "Mimi" Clarke Secor

Thank you to Mimi Secor for the wonderful opportunity to contribute to this project. I am forever grateful to my patients, colleagues, and co-workers, who have provided valuable stories, shared life experiences, and taught me to challenge myself and never stop learning. I would especially like to acknowledge Dr. Joellen Hawkins for being a lifelong mentor and friend. I appreciate the unconditional love, support, and strength from my family, including my husband John and my children Andrew, Amelia, and Evan.

Heidi Collins Fantasia

Introduction
to the Gynecologic Exam

Conducting a gynecologic exam requires many clinical skills. These include competence in establishing and building emotional rapport with patients; knowing how and what questions to ask to elicit an appropriate gynecologic history; conducting a systematic, thorough, accurate pelvic exam in a confident, reassuring manner; and documenting medical records appropriately. Frequently, this involves the use of electronic medical records, including transmitting prescriptions electronically.

I

Conducting the Interview and Taking a Gynecologic and Sexual History

INTRODUCTION

The gynecologic exam visit involves many competencies, skills, and steps, including taking a gynecologic history, conducting a gynecologic exam, excellent communication and clinical skills, and the ability to formulate a management plan to address preventive goals and health issues pertinent to the individual patient. This process is complex and individualized to each patient and situation. Knowledge, practice, and experience are required to develop basic competency and, with time, expert skills.

In this chapter you will learn how to:

1. Develop skills and strategies for creating a therapeutic environment for conducting a gynecologic exam.
2. Obtain key elements of a gynecologic history.
3. Take a gynecologic history, including how to ask questions particularly related to taking a sexual history.

CREATING A THERAPEUTIC ENVIRONMENT

The environment that welcomes the patient into the office set-ting establishes the stage for a therapeutic environment. There are many elements to take into consideration when designing and furnishing a waiting room or area. For example, introduc-ing "comfort" measures into the waiting area communicates that the patient is expected and welcomed. These measures can include comfortable chairs, current magazines, pleasant art on the walls, and access to a water cooler with disposable cups, which can each contribute to increasing the patient's feeling of being welcomed and comfortable upon arrival. Be sure to train the reception personnel to be pleasant, call the patient by name, provide easy instructions for completing needed paperwork, and offer directions to the bathroom, all of which can contribute to a more relaxed patient.

PREAPPOINTMENT INSTRUCTIONS

Before the appointment, the patient should be advised to avoid intravaginal medications, douching, and intercourse within 24 hours of her visit. This improves diagnostic accuracy by minimizing disruptions in the vaginal ecosystem potentially caused by these factors.

ESTABLISHING RAPPORT

It is important to establish and maintain effective rapport with patients and to incorporate various approaches to facili-tate this process. This begins by introducing yourself to each patient by your full name and clearly stating your professional title, nurse practitioner.

FAST FACTS in a NUTSHELL

Always shake the patient's hand (perhaps not during "flu season"). This establishes physical contact, respect, friendliness, and equality. This is the first opportunity for body contact (a gradual approach is good) and is an important component of the gynecologic examination.

Other strategies to help establish rapport include the following:

Professional Image

Dress professionally and wear a nametag in a visible location on your lab coat, scrubs, or clothing. Your nametag should be clearly visible. Some clinicians opt not to wear a lab coat; if you choose to wear street clothes, these should be appropriate to your setting, community, and patient population; always clean and wrinkle free; and communicate a professional image.

The Initial Conversation

Help the patient feel comfortable by asking about her occupation and family and how her day is going. At first glance this may seem like small talk, but it provides both the patient and the clinician with useful information and helps transition into the reason for the patient's visit. This initial conversation helps establish rapport, breaks the ice, and sets the tone for the visit and relationship.

Communicate About the Role of the Nurse Practitioner

Ask if the woman has seen a nurse practitioner before; this can create an opportunity to educate the patient about nurse practitioners, including discussion about your particular specialty, position in the practice, experience, and expertise. You might want to discuss how patients can address you, for example, Mrs. Secor or Ms. Secor or by first name, Mimi. You can also ask the patient, particularly if she is older than you, how she would like to be addressed, by first name or by marital status and last name.

Use Humor

Use appropriate humor to help the patient relax, For example, saying something like, "Men don't know what courage is; it's making a gyn exam appointment and keeping it!" This helps create a moment of levity and bonding. Do, however, avoid inappropriate humor.

INTRODUCTION TO DOCUMENTING THE GYNECOLOGIC EXAM

The Electronic Medical Record (EMR)

Advantages of using an EMR includes enhanced accuracy of documentation and greater opportunity for patients to participate in and negotiate the specific data that are recorded (medicolegal implications). Also, when the clinician becomes proficient, EMR use can actually improve efficiency.

When using EMRs during the interview, position the computer to facilitate optimal eye contact with the patient and to promote ergonomic comfort for both the patient and clinician. Inform the patient that it may be necessary to periodically interrupt the conversation to accurately record findings during the visit. This requires a certain level of proficiency; otherwise, the patient may feel that the clinician is not fully listening to her. Predesigned EMR templates facilitate communications, provide a systematic structure for the work-up, ensure inclusion of the key elements of the assessment, and potentially save time.

Examples of documenting a gynecologic exam visit are provided in sections throughout the next few chapters, as the gynecologic exam is described.

FAST FACTS in a NUTSHELL

Documenting as you progress through the patient visit increases accuracy of data reporting and improves proficiency of EMR use.

INTRODUCTION TO CONDUCTING THE MEDICAL INTERVIEW

Conduct the initial interview in a private location, with the patient fully clothed, and with both you and the patient sitting in relatively close proximity. Inform the patient that the conversation and care are confidential per the Health Insurance Portability and Accountability Act of 1996 ("HIPAA") and that questions you ask are for the purpose of helping to provide the highest quality individualized care, including diagnosis and management of the patient's problems. Note the general appearance of the patient as you conduct the interview and prepare to examine the patient.

Obtain the General Medical History

Elicit a general medical history, being careful to include the following elements:

- Current medical history, including review of systems (ROS)
- Past medical and surgical history
- Family history
- Allergies to medications
- Medications, including nonprescription and over-the-counter; herbs; homeopathics; and supplements
- Health maintenance, such as last Pap smear, mammogram, colonoscopy, bone density, etc.
- Vaccination status
- Social history
  - Occupation, work, home, family, friend network, spiritual base, leisure activities
  - Smoking, alcohol use, recreational drug use
  - Exercise, sleep, stress, diet, nutritional status
  - Abuse history
  - Safe sex practices
  - Distracted driving, seat belts

Obtain the Gynecologic History

Begin the gynecologic history by asking about related problems and taking a detailed history of these problems.

The menstrual history includes the following elements:

- Age of menarche
- Cycle interval (approximately 28 days)
- Duration and amount of flow
- Date (first day) of last menstrual period (LMP)
- Associated menstrual symptoms
  - Recent changes in menses
  - Premenstrual symptoms

- Menorrhagia
- Dysmenorrhea (onset, duration, self-management)
- Late or lighter menses (suspect pregnancy) and associated pregnancy symptoms
- History of unprotected intercourse since LMP (must rule out pregnancy)

FAST FACTS in a NUTSHELL

If the patient reports unprotected intercourse, inconsistent use of birth control, or a later, lighter menses, you must rule out pregnancy. This is especially important if the patient is complaining of pregnancy symptoms, such as breast tenderness, urinary frequency, and/or nausea.

Ask the patient about menstrual history since menarche, being careful to obtain details about the occurrence of:

- Amenorrhea
- Oligomenorrhea
- Pregnancy
- Irregular or abnormal vaginal bleeding (ABV); formerly known as dysfunctional uterine bleeding (DUB)
- Spotting

FAST FACTS in a NUTSHELL

- A history of irregular menses since menarche, especially if there is significant irregularity (skipping months numerous times over one or more years), should prompt you to consider polycystic ovarian syndrome (PCOS).
- Significant dysmenorrhea and dyspareunia over months and/or years may suggest endometriosis or pelvic inflammatory disease (PID).

Obtain Sexual History

Sexual history is a key component of a gynecologic history. How you ask questions and create an environment conducive to disclosure are both critically important factors in taking a sexual history. As a clinician you must help patients feel comfortable discussing their sexuality. Also, you need to take care in avoiding a heterosexual bias.

- Ask about past and current sexual activity.
- Note age of first intercourse, also referred to as "coitarche."
- Estimate the total number of sexual partners the patient has been involved with (including genders and percent of condom use). This information helps you as the clinician to evaluate the patient's risk for cervical cancer and other sexually transmitted infections (STIs).
- If the patient is currently sexually active, ask if her partner is male or female, if she has more than one partner, and if the patient and/or her partners are having sex with men, women, or both.
- Note the duration of the current relationship, along with the date of last intercourse, or sexual relations.
- Ask if the relationship is monogamous; this is critical, as this information helps you to assess STI risk and the need for STI testing.
- Even though the patient may not currently have a sexual partner, she may still be sexually active; ask about utilization of sex toys or other forms of self-stimulation, including masturbation.
- Ask about specific sexual practices, including a history of penile/vaginal intercourse, oral/genital receptive sex, and/or anal receptive intercourse.
- Ask about condom use and estimate the percent of condom use; both are critical to assessing STI and pregnancy risk.

- Elicit and note past or current history of STIs, including both the type and dates of infections, treatment (if known), and any complications or sequelae such as chronic pelvic pain or infertility.
- Ascertain the date when the patient was last tested for STIs, including specific tests and the results. If the patient has current symptoms of a possible STI or vaginitis, elicit a history of present illness, including chief complaint, symptoms, and associated symptoms.

Pap Smear History

Obtain the patient's Pap smear history, as this is critical when evaluating current and past Pap smear results and is important when determining appropriate frequency of screening intervals.

- Ask for date of most recent Pap smear and the results.
- Obtain patient report of abnormal Pap smears in the past, including the dates, any follow-up such as colposcopy and biopsies, and follow-up Pap results.
- Follow the new cervical cancer screening guidelines that recommend the first Pap smear test be conducted at age 21, every 3 years until age 30, then every 5 years.
- Advise patients that they may consider discontinuing Pap screenings after age 65.

History of Urinary Tract Infections

Elicit a history of urinary tract infections (UTIs), including current symptoms, past infections, total number of infections, history of genitourinary surgery or diagnostic tests such as cystoscopy, or urodynamic testing. Asking about a history of urinary tract symptoms or infections is an important part of the gynecologic history because these problems may be associated with gynecologic conditions such as vaginitis or STIs such as genital herpes. UTIs may also be caused by or aggravated by intercourse and/or atrophic vaginitis.

Contraceptive History

Taking a comprehensive contraceptive history is also a key component of the gynecologic history. Include questions about:

- The patient's current contraceptive method, if any
- Level of satisfaction with the method
- Compliance with the method
- Side effects experienced
- Elicit patient questions/concerns about current method
- Ask about past methods used and level of satisfaction or problems associated with these methods
- Unplanned pregnancies, complications, side effects, and other patient concerns

FAST FACTS in a NUTSHELL

A personal or family history, especially of cardiovascular problems, stroke, migraines with aura, or coagulopathies, is important to elicit, especially if the patient is considering combination contraceptives.

ASSESS VITAL SIGNS

Assess specific vital signs based on the reason for the visit and the nature of the patient complaint and clinical problem. If the patient has presented for a well-woman exam, it is reasonable and appropriate to assess full vital signs, including blood pressure, heart rate, weight, body mass index, and height. If a patient has presented for a problem such as vaginitis, it may not be necessary or appropriate to assess full vital signs. However, whenever a patient complains of fever, significant abdominal pain, malaise, or urinary tract symptoms, it is appropriate and essential to assess temperature, blood pressure, and heart rate as well. During this part of the patient interview, you will begin to determine exam components to perform based on the patient's vital signs.

Patient Weight

Assess the patient's weight during a well-woman visit and when indicated based on history. If you note or the patient reports a significant change, assessing weight is even more important. During any visit, patients may ask to have their weight checked regardless of the type of visit, problem based or a periodic well-woman visit.

Vital Signs

1. Assess blood pressure when the woman reports any or all of the following symptoms:
   • Significant abdominal pain
   • Abnormal vaginal bleeding
   • Dizziness
   • Weakness

Promptly assess the patient's blood pressure if you suspect PID, tubal pregnancy, or abnormal vaginal bleeding, or if the patient appears pale, weak, disoriented, diaphoretic, septic, or very ill or in significant pain. Include assessment of heart rate and respiratory rate in each of these clinical situations.

2. Assess heart and respiratory rates:
   • As part of a well-woman exam
   • During problem visits as indicated
   • If the patient appears ill or has constitutional symptoms, or you suspect a significant infection, assessing heart rate is appropriate
   • If the patient reports heart or respiratory problems or complaints
3. Assess the patient's temperature in any of the following clinical situations:
   • Urinary tract symptoms
   • Abdominal pain, especially lower or flank areas
   • Pain with intercourse
   • Vaginal discharge or vaginitis complaints
   • Abnormal vaginal bleeding, irregular or heavy menses

======================*FAST FACTS in a NUTSHELL*

Assess the patient's temperature after the gynecologic exam, especially if you suspect PID even with only mild tenderness on examination of the uterus and/or adnexal area.

Performing additional non–gynecologic examination components is determined by the purpose of visit, patient's complaints, problems, and findings from other aspects of the physical exam performed thus far.

TRANSITIONING TO CONDUCTING THE GYNECOLOGIC EXAM

On completion of the patient interview and obtaining the patient's gynecologic and sexual history, you'll begin to transition to the actual gynecologic exam. Ask the patient to empty her bladder before the examination and collect a urine sample for testing, if indicated. Testing may include a urine dipstick screen, urinalysis, culture, pregnancy test, and STI testing.

In general, conduct the nongynecologic aspects of the physical exam before the gynecologic exam. This helps the patient become comfortable with the clinician. When conducting the physical examination, we recommend a head-to-toe sequence. There may be exceptions in which the clinician and/or the patient prefers to proceed to the gynecologic exam, such as a history of vulvovaginitis, extreme anxiety, sexual abuse, patient requests, or other specific considerations. We will discuss these special situations in more detail in Part II.

2

Abdominal Exam

INTRODUCTION

Performing a thorough abdominal exam is recommended as part of most gynecologic exams, regardless of the patient complaint or reason for the visit, and is included as part of a well-woman exam. Findings derived from this exam provide valuable information to assist you in making an appropriate diagnostic assessment. Both reassuringly normal and abnormal clinical findings of concern can be elicited from performing a thorough abdominal exam. These may include changes in bowel sounds, tenderness (especially rebound), and palpable masses.

In this chapter you will learn:

1. The indications for performing an abdominal exam focusing on urogynecologic complaints.
2. The technique and sequence for performing the abdominal exam.
3. Normal versus abnormal exam findings (Table 2.1).

TABLE 2.1 Assessment Findings of the Abdomen: Normal and Abnormal

Findings of Area Assessed

Normal	Abnormal
Contour and shape are symmetrical, no distention, peristalsis is present	Distention may indicate fibroid tumor, pregnancy, or other masses.
Umbilicus is normal location and skin color	Periumbilical ecchymosis (Cullen's sign) is a classic sign of ruptured ectopic pregnancy. Spider angiomas, commonly associated with pregnancy, appear just above the umbilicus between the second and fifth months.
Skin is blemish free and may be lightly covered with hair	Rashes; lesions such as pruritic urticarial papules of pregnancy (PUPP) appear as coalescing papules on the abdomen (rarely near the umbilicus) during the last trimester and resolve postpartum; burns may indicate abuse; scars should be investigated related to past surgeries, including hysterectomies.
Diastasis recti muscle should be smooth and firm	Separation of the abdominal rectus muscles (results of pregnancy, multiparity, congenital weakness, marked obesity)
Presence of striae (linea alba) is common from skin stretched during pregnancy	Purple lines may suggest Cushing's disease.
Palpation of lower abdomen is normally nontender and pain free	Tenderness in presence of reported pelvic pain suggests PID, ectopic pregnancy, ovarian cyst, or urinary tract infection. Tenderness may also suggest appendicitis, esp. if right lower quadrant.
Inguinal lymph nodes are soft, mobile, and nontender	Enlarged, soft, and tender nodes indicate STIs such as herpes simplex virus. Hard, irregular, immobile nodes require referral to a specialist.

18

(continued)

TABLE 2.1 *(continued)*

Findings of Area Assessed	
Normal	**Abnormal**
Bowel sounds	Absence of bowel sounds may suggest acute abdomen, obstruction, ruptured appendicitis, etc. Increased bowel sounds may be present with PID, gastrointestinal infections/conditions, and sepsis.

Adapted from Carcio, H. A., & Secor, M. C. (2010). *Advanced health assessment of women: Clinical skills and procedures* (2nd ed., pp. 67–69). New York, NY: Springer Publishing Company; and Rhoads, J. (2006). *Advanced health assessment and diagnostic reasoning* (pp. 277, 332). Philadelphia, PA: Lippincott Williams & Wilkins.

The abdominal examination should precede the gynecologic examination, as it provides clues to the nature of the patient complaint and may also reduce patient anxiety associated with anticipating the gynecologic examination. This may not be the case if the patient has a history of sexual abuse (see Chapter 8).

Indications for a gynecologic exam focusing on urogynecologic complaints include:

- Constitutional symptoms: fever, chills, malaise, nausea, vomiting
- Urinary tract symptoms
- Abdominal pain, especially in lower or flank areas
- Dyspareunia (pain with intercourse)
- Vaginal discharge
- Abnormal vaginal bleeding, irregular or heavy menses
- Missed, late menses
- Post exam as indicated, especially if you suspect pelvic inflammatory disease (PID), even with mild tenderness on examination of the uterus and adnexae

You do not need to wear gloves during the abdominal exam unless the woman has open or moist lesions or if the lower abdominal exam involves assessing the upper genital area. This includes the groin, mons, and suprapublic areas.

Position the patient in a supine or low semi-Fowler's position while you, the examiner, stand on the patient's right side. This is not always possible depending on the layout of the examination room. Throughout the exam, closely monitor the woman's facial expressions for signs of discomfort and evidence of anxiety. This is particularly important when assessing severity of pain or tenderness reported during the history.

If the patient is in severe discomfort (even at rest), she is likely to be unable to lie on the exam table in a fully supine position with her legs extended flat on the exam table. She may prefer to bend her knees and may not be able to lay still or concentrate on the conversation or examination. Note if she appears to be in mild, moderate, or severe distress. Also observe if she appears pale, apprehensive, diaphoretic, weak, withdrawn, restless, or uncooperative.

Washing your hands in front of the patient just prior to commencing the exam is a good practice and serves both to consistently maintain a clean environment and to reassure the patient. Researchers have demonstrated that patients feel more confident with clinicians who wash their hands in front of them.

FAST FACTS in a NUTSHELL

If the woman is ticklish, it may be helpful to start the examination by placing the patient's hand under or on top of your examination hand.

If the patient complains of urinary tract symptoms, it is important to assess for pyelonephritis by checking for costovertebral angle tenderness (CVAT), particularly if associated constitutional symptoms such as fever, chills, weakness, nausea, or vomiting are noted.

To assess for CVAT, stand behind the patient, placing the palm of one hand over the lateral aspect of patient's mid thoracic area. With the fist of the other hand, gently hit the top of the hand placed on the patient's back. If this maneuver causes patient discomfort, the test is considered a positive for CVA tenderness, indicating possible pyelonephritis.

If the patient is complaining of abdominal pain, it is essential to perform a thorough abdominal exam. The order of the abdominal exam is as follows:

1. Observation/inspection
2. Auscultation for bowel sounds
3. Percussion for abnormal air, masses, liver, spleen, costovertebral tenderness
4. Light palpation for tenderness, including rebound (pain after releasing pressure)
5. Deeper palpation for liver, masses, and unusual tenderness

1. Observe/inspect: Begin the abdominal exam with observation.
   - Inspect for asymmetry and abdominal distention.
   - Note any scars that may include surgical or abuse scars, rashes, or lesions.
   - Observe for Cullen's sign (ecchymosis around the umbilicus, ruptured ectopic pregnancy, or intraperitoneal bleeding).
   - Grey-Turner's sign (ecchymosis in flank area)—may indicate previous abdominal trauma or abuse.
2. Next, auscultate the abdomen for bowel sounds in all four quadrants.
   - Note sounds as normal, absent, abnormally loud bowel sounds (referred to as borborygmi).
   - Sounds may be high-pitched (normal small intestine) or low-pitched and rumbling (large intestine).
   - Lack of bowel sounds may suggest an obstruction, while abnormally loud bowel sounds—borborygmi—may indicate some other type of gastrointestinal problem.

3. Percuss the abdomen by placing your middle finger on the abdomen and tapping over the tip of that finger with the middle finger of the other hand.
    • High-pitched sounds might suggest a distended abdomen.
    • Dull sounds might suggest enlarged organs or mass(es).
    • Palpate, first lightly using the palm of your hand, then deeper using palmer surfaces of extended fingers, applying firm pressure with second hand on top to deliver deeper pressure. Include assessment of possible rebound tenderness.
    • Goal of light palpation is to assess areas of reported pain or tenderness.
    • Examine the quadrant in which pain has been reported last, to avoid tensing of muscles.
    • Rebound tenderness is defined as the patient describing more pain upon release of the palpation.
    • Note Fast Facts caution (below).
4. For complaints of lower abdominal pain or unusual tenderness in a female, it is important to consider a range of causes in the differential diagnosis, including:
    • Urinary tract infection
    • PID
    • Pregnancy, especially ectopic
    • Ovarian cysts
    • Cancer
    • Vaginitis
    • STIs
    • Gastrointestinal causes
    • Appendicitis
    • Muscle strain
    • Trauma

====*FAST FACTS in a NUTSHELL*

If you suspect severe pain or a mass, do not deeply palpate, as this may cause rupture of an ovarian cyst or ectopic pregnancy or appendicitis.

3

Vulvar Exam

INTRODUCTION

Performing a comprehensive assessment of the female external genitalia requires knowledge of the anatomy, involving the patient, and using a systemic approach to carefully observe and palpate the various tissues and anatomic features. Examining the vulvar region provides the opportunity to detect anatomic changes and other abnormal physical examination findings that may provide diagnostic clues about the possible diagnosis of any patient symptoms described during the patient interview.

In this chapter you will learn how to:

1. Describe the anatomy of the external genitalia, including key structures and landmarks.
2. Conduct a systematic assessment of the external genitalia.
3. Describe normal and abnormal external genitalia findings.

THE APPROACH

After helping the patient assume the lithotomy position, offer the patient a self-examination mirror. We prefer an adjustable telescoping mirror that allows patient viewing without interfering as the clinician conducts the examination. Some general strategies that help to reduce patient anxiety include:

1. Obtaining the patient's permission before proceeding with the exam.
2. Explaining the steps involved in the exam and what the patient can expect to experience. This provides the patient with anticipatory guidance, education, and support.
3. Answering questions as they arise; describing normal and abnormal findings to the patient is educational and often empowering.
4. Wearing gloves throughout the gynecologic exam and when handling any equipment, supplies, or specimens.
5. Using a cotton, Dacron, or new vaginal pH swab (VS-Sense) as a pointer to educate the patient about normal and abnormal anatomy and findings. This same swab may be used to separate skin folds and to assess for tenderness and allodynia (abnormal tenderness or pain to light touch).
6. After the exam, don new gloves while handling lab specimens, including Pap smears, sexually transmitted infection (STI) (Table 3.1), and vaginal microscopy specimens.

FAST FACTS in a NUTSHELL

Some authorities recommend double gloving, then after performing the vulvar exam (Table 3.2), removing the outer glove in order to maintain an uncontaminated environment. When in doubt, it is better to change gloves than to risk contamination.

TABLE 3.1 Sexually Transmitted Infection Assessment of the Female

Infection + Cause	Prevalence	Symptoms	Diagnosis
Chancroid *Haemophilus ducreyi*, gram-negative bacillus	More common in sex trade	Women often asymptomatic	Culture + for *H. ducreyi*, rule out more common HSV, also HIV, syphilis by RPR
Chlamydia Obligate intracellular parasite susceptible to antibiotics	Most common reported STI, 3 million new cases a year	Women often asymptomatic	Universal screening if <26 years old; urine polymerase chain reaction (PCR) or cervical testing; vaginal testing PCR or NAAT testing both approved
Genital Herpes Type 1 or 2 herpes virus: Both can infect genitals	Estimated 55 million Americans infected	Most asymptomatic: symptoms may include painful genital lesions, first infection most severe, recurrences most common with HSV 2, widely variable symptoms	Classic symptoms suspect HSV. Culture if lesions, PCR culture more sensitive, expensive; type-specific serology IGG/HerpeSelect, 98% seroconversion 4 months post-HSV acquisition
Genital Warts Nononcogenic HPV 6, 11	1 million visits yearly, HPV affecting up to 80% of sexually active young women in US	Single or multiple, soft, fleshy, nontender, cauliflower-like lesions in genital area (vulvovaginal, anal, or cervix)	By exam, RPR to rule out condylomata lata of syphilis; colposcopy and/or biopsy of atypical lesions
Gonorrhea *Neisseria gonorrhoeae*, gram-negative diplococcus bacteria	Second most common STI in US, especially among men having sex with men (MSM)	Women commonly asymptomatic, or abnormal vaginal discharge, dysuria, abnormal menses	Gram stain, culture, NAAT of cervical secretions; urine NAAT an option, too; vaginal NAAT for oro-pharyngeal testing

(continued)

TABLE 3.1 Sexually Transmitted Infection Assessment of the Female (continued)

Infection + Cause	Prevalence	Symptoms	Diagnosis
Pelvic Inflammatory Disease (PID) Polymicrobial, various combinations, *N. gonorrhoeae*, *C. trachomatis*, anaerobes, and others	1 million new cases yearly, leading cause of female infertility	Many have no or atypical symptoms. Symptoms include pain/tenderness lower abdomen, uterus, ovaries, fever, chills, and elevated WBCs/erythrocyte sedimentation rate (ESR) associated with menses	High index of suspicion, low threshold for diagnosis, positive cultures, Centers for Disease Control and Prevention criteria, pelvic exam tenderness, mucopus, WBCs on vaginal microscopy, gonorrhea, chlamydia or anaerobes/facultative bacteria
Syphilis *Treponema palladium* spirochete	Increasing among MSM, unusual in women, unless risk factors, higher rates in sex workers (SW)	Primary: classic chancre is painless, indurated ulcer in genital area, may evade diagnosis if vaginal Secondary: variable skin rash, may involve palmar hands, soles of feet Latent: few clinical symptoms, CNS changes	Primary: darkfield exam of chancre, with RPR serology Secondary/latent: RPR serology
Trichomoniasis Motile protozoan	Most common curable STI, 3 million US women infected yearly. May be asymptomatic for years	Excessive, frothy, yellow-green vaginal discharge, exam findings variable, sometimes with genital erythema, swelling, and pruritus	Vaginal microscopy for typical motile trichomonads and WBCs; Pap should be verified with culture or microscopy Various vaginal cultures may also be used

Adapted with permission from Carcio, H. A., & Secor, M. C. (2010). *Advanced health assessment of women: Clinical skills and procedures* (2nd ed., pp. 340–342). New York, NY: Springer Publishing Company.

TABLE 3.2 Assessment of the Vulvar Region External Genitalia

Normal Findings of Area Assessed	Abnormal: List Findings, Then Conditions; Need to Be Consistent
Vulva	LESIONS: biopsy if new, changing or suspicious, or persisting beyond 6 to 8 weeks (general guideline)
Labia majora—hair covered	Small nontender, nonpigmented nodules (Fordyce spots, normal variant, usually within Hart's line, inner labia)
Labia minora—pink, moist, shiny	Nontender, firm, larger nodules (sebaceous cysts)
Butterfly wing shape bilaterally	Large, tender, swollen lump at 5 or 7 o'clock of introitus (Bartholin cyst)
	Single-stalk, finger-like fimbrillations, inner labia (micropapillomatosis labialis, considered normal variant)
	Cauliflower-like growths, usually nontender (genital warts)
	Round, firm, umbilicated nontender papules (molluscum contagiousum)
	Ulcer, nontender, non/well-demarcated/border (chancre of primary syphilis or chancroid)
	Single/clustered, tender vesicles or ulcerations (genital herpes, cellulitis, MRSA, hydradenitis suppurativa, trichomoniasis ulcers, HIV ulcers)
	Irregular, nontender, lesions; pigmented, red, or white (vulvar carcinoma/vulvar intraepithelial neoplasia [VIN], precancer)
	Scarring (genital mutilation/cutting, Crohn's, episiotomy, etc.)
	Distended blood vessels, tender, often in clusters (varicosities usually pregnancy related)
	Fissures; thin, tender, longitudinal (may be associated with infections [i.e., yeast or genital herpes], inflammation [i.e., allergic/contact reactions], skin conditions [i.e., lichen sclerosis (LS)], lichen simplex chronicus [LSC])
	Fissures; large, tender, "knife-like lesions" (Crohn's disease)

(continued)

27

TABLE 3.2 Assessment of the Vulvar Region External Genitalia (continued)

Normal Findings of Area Assessed	Abnormal: List Findings, Then Conditions; Need to Be Consistent
	REDNESS/ERYTHEMA/TENDERNESS Inflammation (seborrheic dermatitis, psoriasis, eczema, lichen planus [LP], allergens, irritants such as soaps, detergents, dryer sheets, chlorine) Infection (*Candida*, trichomoniasis, fungal, bacterial) Focal erythema may be associated with genital herpes, vestibulodynia if within the introital area/vestibule May be associated with acute, chronic vaginitis, or may be idiopathic DISCOLORATION OR PIGMENTATION Dark or pigmented lesions (usually benign; but nevi can develop into melanoma); biopsy new, very dark, large, changing, or symptomatic lesions to rule out melanoma and other cancers/precancers White or hypopigmented areas (LS; squamous hyperplasia, also known as LSC, or possibly VIN) BRUISES (consider possible sexual assault) ANATOMIC CHANGES ASSOCIATED WITH SKIN CONDITIONS Flattening of the posterior labia minora (early LP) Loss of landmarks (LS, LP), agglutination (LS), flattening of labia (LS, LP), parchment-like changes (LS), tenderness, whitening (LS, LP, LSC, must biopsy to clarify diagnosis and to rule out VIN, infection, irritant, contact, atrophy)
Clitoris Round, pink erectile tissue underneath the clitoral hood; Size = approximately 2 cm (0.75 inch) × 0.5 cm (0.195 inch)	ENLARGEMENT Masculinizing conditions (excess testosterone; use of testosterone-containing medications) ATROPHY May virtually disappear (LS)

Urethral Meatus
Pink tissue without discharge

CARUNCLE—small protrusion through the orifice that resembles a polyp (estrogen deprivation)

PROLAPSE OF URETHRAL MUCOSA—presents as a swollen red ring around the urinary meatus (menopause)

LEAKING OF URINE—stress, urge, mixed incontinence

Vaginal Introitus
Small amount of white to clear discharge
Intact hymen or hymenal tags/tissues
No bulging
No redness, lesions, tenderness, normal

DISCHARGE (vaginitis; cervicitis)

THICK, PINK MEMBRANE (imperforate hymen)

ANTERIOR BULGING (cystocele; may be aggravated by obesity)

POSTERIOR BULGING (rectocele, enterocele)

Focal erythema and tenderness at 5 and/or 7 o'clock (vestibulodynia)

Allodynia (suggests vestibulodynia)

Leaking of urine or feces (vaginal fistula)

Perineum and Anus
Skin between vaginal introitus and anus should appear pink, smooth

SCAR—episiotomy

SKIN TAGS

FISSURES

Erythema (vulvovaginitis)

Focal erythema in fourchette (vestibulodynia)

HEMORRHOIDS

Adapted with permission from Carcio, H. A., & Secor, M. C. (2010). *Advanced health assessment of women: Clinical skills and procedures* (2nd ed., pp. 67–69). New York, NY: Springer Publishing Company.

EXTERNAL EXAMINATION OF THE GENITALIA

The systematic approach to examining the external genitalia (Figure 3.1) includes an initial visual examination followed by palpation and separation of skin folds; assessment for tenderness, masses, muscle tension, or any other abnormal findings.

The systematic steps in the external examination include:

- Visually inspecting the suprapubic area, visualizing superiorly to inferiorly and then laterally.
- Inspecting the mons pubis for condition of skin and pubic hair or presence of lesions, masses, foreign bodies such as pubic lice, and/or tenderness.
- Assessing the clitoral hood, clitoris, urethral meatus, Skene's ducts adjacent to the urethral meatus, and the vaginal introitus.
- Carefully examining the hymenal tissues, labia minora, labia majora, perineum, rectum, and sacrum areas.
- Inspecting and gently palpating the upper inner thighs, buttocks, and lower back depending on the patient's history and symptoms.

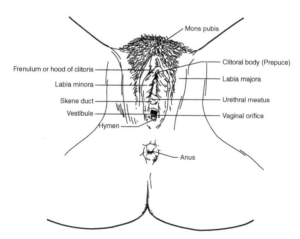

FIGURE 3.1   External genitalia (with revised labels; from Carcio & Secor [2010], Figure 1.1, p. 4).

FOCUS OF THE VISUAL EXAMINATION

Observe the vaginal introitus. The labia minora normally are shaped like butterfly wings. In early lichen planus, there may be flattening or an absence of the lower posterior aspects of the labia minora. These findings may be symmetrical or asymmetrical. Observe for appearance of a cystocele (bulging or herniation of the bladder into the vagina and introitus) or rectocele (bulging of the rectum into the floor of the vagina).

Locate Hart's line, which is the mucocutaneous border separating the inner labia minora (pink, moist, thin, no hair) from the more keratinized skin lateral to the inner labia minora (normal skin color, thicker, hair covered). Hart's line extends superiorly to the clitoris and inferiorly to the perineum. Most patients with vulvovaginitis are most symptomatic medial to Hart's line.

Identify the hymenal area—an imperforate hymen is a continuous membranous "fold" covering the vaginal introitus; a perforated hymen appears as multiple overlapping skin flaps along the margins of the introitus (these are sometimes called hymen caruncles). A hymen that appears imperforated (intact) is common in young girls and in virginal women.

Observe for abnormal findings in the genital area that may include redness, swelling, tenderness, loss of landmarks, masses, foreign bodies such as pubic lice, lesions (such as vesicles, papules, or rashes), fissures, scarring, whitening, abnormal dark pigmented lesions, agglutination of skin folds (the examiner should be able to separate skin folds), and absence of normal hair distribution.

Note any clinical signs indicating possible dermatologic conditions, including lesions, infections, or other abnormalities. Many clinicians and patients assume most vulvovaginal complaints are related to "yeast," candida, or monilial infections. However, there are many non-yeast causes of vulvovaginal complaints, including vaginal causes (STIs, BV, atrophic changes), vulvar dermatologic conditions (lichen simplex chronicus, lichen sclerosis, lichen planus, sensitive skin and conditions secondary to numerous possible external irritants), hygienic practices, and, less commonly, allergens.

Patient Education Tips: General vulvar self-care guidelines you can use to educate patients are described in Appendix D.

Common STIs include the following:

- Chlamydia
- Herpes simplex (Figure 3.2a)
- Condylomata (genital warts; Figure 3.2b)
- Gonorrhea
- Pelvic inflammatory disease (PID)
- Syphilis
- Chancroid

To complete the visual exam, palpation is required to separate skin folds, identify hidden clinical findings, and palpate any areas of erythema, masses, or other abnormal skin findings. Palpation detects masses and tenderness not otherwise identified by inspection alone, such as Bartholin's gland cysts (Figure 3.3a,b). Use a cotton or Dacron swab to localize and grade tenderness and to assess for allodynia (abnormal sensation).

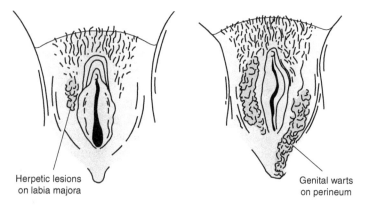

Herpetic lesions
on labia majora

Genital warts
on perineum

FIGURE 3.2 (a) Genital herpes, (b) Genital warts.

FAST FACTS in a NUTSHELL

Allodynia is the perception of tenderness or pain with light palpation in an area that is not normally painful when touched lightly with a gloved finger or a small swab. Allodynia may be associated with acute or chronic vulvar pain and/or vestibulodynia, vaginismus, and, less commonly, some dermatologic conditions such as lichen planus or lichen sclerosis.

PALPATION

After completing the visual inspection of the vaginal introitus, separate the tissue fragments of the hymen (looking for focal erythema or lesions) and folds of the labia. Palpate the introitus for tenderness or masses focusing on the Bartholin's gland duct areas, which are located at 5 and 7 o'clock. Bartholin's glands should be smooth and nontender. Tenderness on palpation or presence of a mass requires follow-up. If tenderness is elicited, the location is recorded as if the introitus is a face of a clock (erythema at 3 o'clock) and the severity of tenderness rated on a scale of 1 to 10 (with 10 representing the most severe pain).

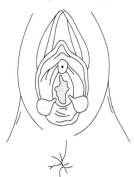

FIGURE 3.3a Bartholin's glands.

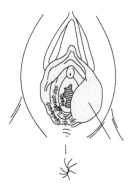

FIGURE 3.3b Bartholin cyst.

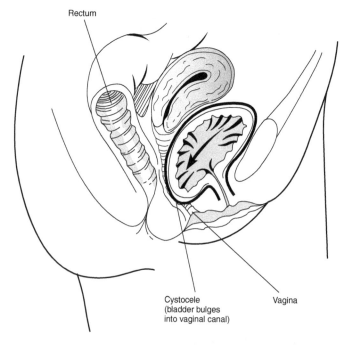

Rectum

Cystocele
(bladder bulges
into vaginal canal)

Vagina

FIGURE 3.4 Cystocele.

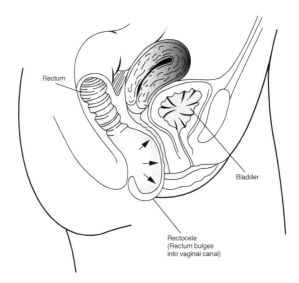

FIGURE 3.5   Rectocele.

Next, assess for vaginal introital tone and vaginismus laxity.

- Abnormal tone may be referred to as hytone dysfunction and may be more marked on one side than the other.
- Vaginismus, the involuntary spasm of the pelvic floor muscles, is usually associated with anxiety and possibly a past history of sexual trauma. Examining a patient with vaginismus can be very challenging and is discussed in Part II.

When evaluating vaginal introital tone, perform the following maneuvers to test for laxity and tone:

1. The test for laxity involves asking the patient to bear down or Valsalva; this may expose a cystocele, bulging of the bladder into the vagina (Figure 3.4), or a rectocele, bulging of the rectum up into the vaginal floor (Figure 3.5).

2. Before and during the Valsalva maneuver, observe for prolapse of the uterus (a descent of the uterus from its normal position into the vagina, and sometimes, out of the body). Uterine prolapse (Figure 3.6) may also be apparent without the pressure placed upon it during Valsalva. If present, note the degree of prolapse from first degree (minimal lowering of cervix into vagina cavity), second degree (where the cervix is visible at the vaginal introitus), third degree (where the cervix is visible outside the vagina), and fourth degree (where the cervix and the uterus are entirely externally prolapsed). This most extreme case is called *procidentia.*

3. The test for introital tone, or hytone dysfunction, involves palpating the introital tissues for abnormal muscle tension/spasm and associated tenderness. Introital tone is also assessed by inserting one finger into the vagina and asking the patient to "tighten" around the examiner's finger. This requires contracting the pubococcygeal (PC) muscle as though the patient is holding her urine and/or bowels.

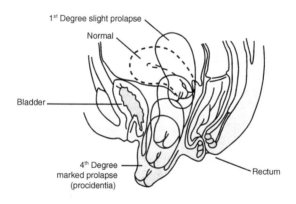

FIGURE 3.6 Degrees of uterine prolapse.

FAST FACTS in a NUTSHELL

A positive "sticky glove test" indicates possible atrophic vaginitis. This test is conducted by lightly palpating the inner labia minora, noting whether your gloved fingers adhere to the tissue. This finding is common in post-menopausal women, due to diminished estrogen production. The finding is subtle and the inexperienced clinician must be attentive to appreciate it. (See Chapter 11 for more information on atrophic vaginitis.)

PELVIC FLOOR REHABILITATION

- Some patients may not be able to isolate the PC muscle. Patients who are experiencing symptoms of overactive bladder (OAB), including urgency, frequency, or leakage; dyspareunia; or chronic vulvar pain may benefit from pelvic floor rehabilitation combined with biofeedback and possibly electrical stimulation (also called E-stim). These exercises help strengthen the pelvic floor (Figure 3.7) and counter detrusor instability associated with OAB, often greatly improving the symptoms of OAB.
- Pelvic floor rehabilitation includes exercises to strengthen the pelvic floor muscles (levator ani and pubococcygeal muscles). These exercises include Kegel's (5–10 seconds) and "quick flick" (5 seconds) exercises.
- Electrical stimulation (E-stim) helps patients isolate and learn how to contract their PC muscle, which is required to perform both Kegel's and "quick flick" exercises.

38

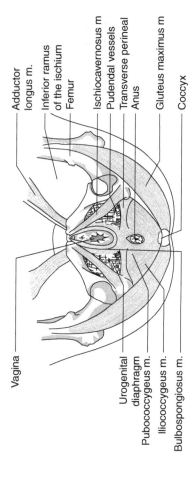

Vagina

Adductor
longus m.

Inferior ramus
of the ischium

Femur

Ischiocavernosus m

Pudendal vessels

Transverse perineal

Anus

Gluteus maximus m

Coccyx

Urogenital
diaphragm

Pubococcygeus m.

Iliococcygeus m.

Bulbospongiosus m.

FIGURE 3.7 Anatomy and musculature of pelvic floor.

4

The Speculum Exam

INTRODUCTION

The purpose of the speculum exam is to visualize the vagina and the cervix. Note both normal findings and abnormalities. The speculum exam also allows you to collect a cervical sample for a Papanicolaou (Pap) smear and to screen for sexually transmitted infections (STIs), as well as vaginitis as indicated. To optimize the results of the testing, the sample must be collected properly.

In this chapter you will learn how to:

1. Prepare for the speculum exam.
2. Select the appropriate speculum for an individual patient.
3. Insert, secure, and remove the speculum.
4. Locate and visualize the cervix and properly obtain a Pap smear.

PREPARING TO PERFORM THE SPECULUM EXAM

Gather the equipment needed to perform the exam:

- A light suitable for illuminating the pelvic area during the exam; consider using a gooseneck light or a light attached to a plastic speculum.

- Vaginal speculum: both plastic and metal are options (see later for the advantages and disadvantages of each)
- Water-soluble lubricant
- Supplies for obtaining the Pap smear and any cultures that may be necessary
- Non-latex gloves

The NEW 2012 Cervical Cancer Screening Guidelines	
Age 21	Screening should begin
Ages 21-29	Cytology alone is recommended every 3 years
Ages 30-65	Co-testing (Pap and HPV) every 5 years is recommended If HPV testing is not available, cytology alone should be continued every 3 years
Age 65	Screening may stop

2012 USPSTF, ACS, ASCCP

PREPARE THE PATIENT FOR WHAT TO EXPECT DURING THE SPECULUM EXAM

The following hints are useful in promoting patient comfort and reducing anxiety (reprinted with permission from Carcio & Secor, 2010, p. 62):

- Offer an educational pelvic examination, by explaining the techniques used, the sensations that the patient may feel, and the function of the body parts examined.
- Explain each aspect of the examination as you perform it, to reduce the woman's level of anxiety. Always be as gentle as possible.

- Explain the rationale for each aspect of the exam and provide clues about what she might "feel"; for example, "You might feel some pressure when I insert my fingers into your vagina"
- Suggest coping strategies to minimize stress your patient might be experiencing:
  - Encourage her to progressively relax different body parts or to try taking deep breaths and exhaling slowly at any point during the exam when she feels especially tense.
  - Teach use of "self-talk" statements such as "I know this may be slightly uncomfortable but I will be fine."
- Reassure her that you will stop at any time that she becomes uncomfortable.

POSITIONING THE PATIENT

The lithotomy position is the traditional position for the vaginal or speculum exam. Assist the patient to slide down to the end of the examination table while providing support by placing your hands at the end of the exam table under the patient's buttocks. This ensures the patient knows when she has reached the end of the table/has slid down far enough, and also helps the patient feel more comfortable and secure. When she is in the correct position, her buttocks should be at the end of the examination table (slightly overhanging), with her heels placed in the stirrups, knees bent, and hips externally rotated and abducted.

Inform the patient prior to inserting the speculum, explaining the procedure and reminding her of the sensations she may experience during each part of the procedure. Ask the patient to inform you at any time of pain or other unpleasant symptoms experienced during the exam, and assure the patient that you will stop if she requests you to do so.

SELECTING THE SPECULUM

Vaginal specula are available in metal and plastic of varying styles, sizes, and quality. Plastic specula come in fewer sizes, styles, and, most important, range in quality. The less expensive plastic specula may not reliably unlock prior to removal. This inability to release the speculum can cause you anxiety and the patient additional anxiety, pain, and possibly injury when you remove the speculum with the blades in an open position. To lessen this risk, you should familiarize yourself with the speculum prior to examining the patient.

The major advantages of metal specula include the following:

- Available in many styles (Pederson, Graves, bariatric, and many others).
- Available in many sizes (small, medium, large, etc.) to accommodate different types of patients and their unique needs, including pediatric, multiparous, obese, and those with physical disabilities.
- Can be prewarmed with tap water, by holding them briefly in your gloved hand, or by placing them on a heating pad (on low setting in the exam table storage drawer) or running the speculum under warm water.
- Can be sterilized for reuse, offering an economical and "green" option.

The major advantages of plastic specula include the following:

- Provide an unobstructed view of the vaginal walls through the clear blades.
- No prewarming the speculum before insertion is required.

- Use may reduce patient anxiety because the clear plastic appearance is less "scary" than metal.
- Some models are designed with plug-in lighting systems (such as Welch Allyn corded or cordless) and offer enhanced illumination and examination of the vagina and cervix.
- Conveniently, this external light source may also be used to examine the vulva prior to speculum insertion.

Unpredictably on occasion, plastic specula can break in-situ or be difficult to "unlock" upon removal. This is potentially traumatic for both the patient and the clinician. If the speculum can't be unlocked then it must be removed with the blades open, which can cause pain and injure the patient's external genitalia. Another disadvantage of plastic specula is their contribution to medical waste because they are not reusable.

Appropriate Speculum Size

To determine the size and type of the speculum, most appropriate for examining a patient, you should evaluate the diameter and tone of the vaginal introitus. Other factors to consider include use of a smaller speculum if the patient is symptomatic or anxious.

Helpful tips to reduce discomfort during the exam include the following:

- Palpate the cervix before inserting the speculum especially if this is the patient's first exam, if the patient is symptomatic, has a history of abuse or trauma, or has experienced "difficult or challenging" exams in the past.
- Use a small amount of lubricant if needed.
- Palpating the cervix in advance of the speculum exam may help in selecting the more appropriate speculum style and/or size.

INSERTING THE SPECULUM

1. Separate the labia minora with your nondominant hand to expose the vaginal opening.
2. Hold the speculum with your dominant hand, grasping in a manner that keeps the blades securely closed. To do this, place your index finger on top of the upper blade near the handle, and your middle finger under the base of the lower blade (where the handle meets the blades). This is the recommended hand position for insertion and removal of the speculum.
3. Holding the speculum at a slight sideways angle, insert the speculum in a downward direction, approximately two inches into the vagina. See Speculum Insertion (Figure 4.1A).
4. Use a gentle side-to-side "shimmy" to advance the speculum.
5. When the speculum is in place, open the speculum by repositioning both hands: one hand controls opening the speculum blades and the other hand holds the lower handle of the speculum. See Speculum Insertion (Figure 4.1B).
6. Once partially visualized, open the speculum more until the cervix pops fully into view (Speculum Insertion, Figure 4.1C). You may have to lift the lower "chin" of the cervix by a further gentle side-to-side "shimmy" of the speculum blades to "coax" the cervix into full view.
7. Secure the speculum by either rotating the metal wheel/knob on the side of the speculum handle or locking the plastic blades together in an open position, just enough to view and sample the cervix.

Potential patient discomfort occurs from tension at the vaginal opening caused by opening of the speculum blades. Larger specula create more tension or stretching of the vaginal opening and potentially more patient discomfort. This

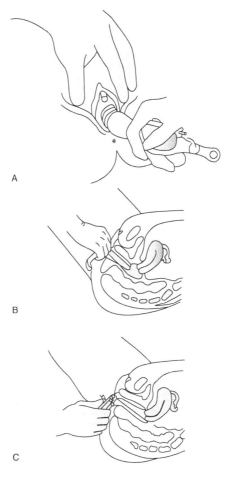

A

B

C

FIGURE 4.1 Speculum insertion.

(**A**) Index finger and thumb on the top, middle, and ring finger below (read how described in text).

(**B**) Turn the speculum so that the blades are horizontal to the examining table as you advance the speculum into the vagina, pressing downward toward with the lower blade on the posterior vaginal wall at a 45-degree angle.

(**C**) Once in place, open the speculum and maneuver the blades until the cervix is visible.

is especially important to appreciate when examining symptomatic patients, those having their first examination, pediatric patients, and any patients with a history of anxiety, vaginismus, dyspareunia, or emotional or physical sexual abuse or pain.

═══════════════════════════*FAST FACTS in a NUTSHELL*

- To examine certain patients who are symptomatic, anxious, or have a history of sexual abuse, it may be necessary to only partially open the speculum blades, while viewing and sampling the cervix as quickly as possible.
- When using a plastic Welch Allyn speculum, take care to lift the adjustment tab (white ratchet) when opening the speculum blades, to avoid causing a loud repetitive clicking sound as the blades are opened. If you do not lift the tab, warn patients to expect this "clicking" sound.

INSPECTING THE VAGINA AND CERVIX

Visualize the vagina for color (normally pink) and rugations, which are vaginal folds normally present in women of reproductive age. You may note a small amount of opaque, white, nonmalodorous discharge. During the visual inspection, you should also note any redness, pallor, lack of rugation, abnormal bulging of the vaginal walls (a cystocele is a bulging of the upper front wall of the vagina, a rectocele is a bulging of the lower rear wall of the vagina, and a enterocele is a bulging of the upper rear wall of the vagina), lesions, abnormal discharge (such as frothy, yellow, or malodorous discharge), lesions, foreign bodies, or other unusual findings (Table 4.1 and Figure 4.2).

TABLE 4.1 Normal and Abnormal Assessment Findings of the Vagina and Cervix

Findings of Area Assessed

Normal	Abnormal
Vagina	
Normally pink Discharge: opaque, white, nonmalodorous mucus emitted from Skene glands Normal pH: acidic	Gonorrhea or Chlamydia: abundance of polymorphonuclear WBCs Vaginal discharge: • Candida vulvovaginitis: thick, white, clumpy discharge • Bacterial vaginosis: thin, fishy odor, coaty white or gray • Trichomoniasis: yellow, grayish-green, frothy, malodorous • Vaginitis: elevated pH, positive amine test, abnormal discharge, erythema, variable (rare vaginally)
Vagina: mucosa Normal: rugae (mucosal folds) negative	Atrophic vaginitis; Thin, pale atrophic-appearing mucosa, variable discharge, scant, copious, watery, yellow or lack of rugae is evidence of low estrogen level • Cystocele; bulging (herniation) of the bladder into the upper front vaginal wall • Rectocele: bulging (herniation) of the rectum into the rear vaginal wall • Enterocele: bulging (herniation) of the small intestine into the upper rear vaginal wall
Cervix	
Size and shape Nulliparous (small and oval or round) Parous (slit-like)	Laceration or tears: may result from a precipitous delivery of baby Tiny os (may also be noted in nulliparous women who are not taking hormone replacement therapy)

(continued)

TABLE 4.1 *(continued)*

Findings of Area Assessed	
Normal	**Abnormal**
Surface: color is pink, smooth, soft, mobile, and nontender on movement	Bluish (cyanotic): associated with pregnancy Tender on movement: may indicate pelvic inflammatory disease Fixed or immobile: may indicate endometriosis or a tumor Polyps: small, red-purple, pedunculated protrusions; typically arising from endocervical canal; more common during menstruating years and in parous women in fifth decade Nabothian cysts: can be single or multiple; small, translucent or yellow nodules on the cervical surface
Mucosa characteristics: intact, no lesions	Friability: may be related to infection such as Chlamydia or vaginitis Wart-like excoriation: may be associated with cervical cancer Extension of endocervical columnar epithelium on the ectocervix (ectropion): evidence of increased estrogen production in pregnancy or effect of birth control pills Erosion: friable tissues surrounding os associated cervicitis
Location	Lower in the vagina: possible uterine prolapse Lowering of more than 3 cm may suggest an ovarian mass

Sources: Carcio & Secor (2010, pp. 81–82); Rhoads (2006, pp. 333, 338).

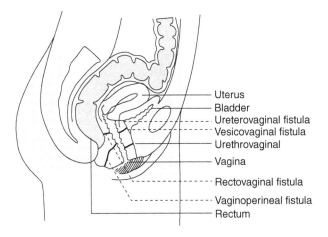

Uterus
Bladder
Ureterovaginal fistula
Vesicovaginal fistula
Urethrovaginal
Vagina
Rectovaginal fistula
Vaginoperineal fistula
Rectum

FIGURE 4.2   Locations of various fistulas.

The cervix is normally pink, smooth, and nontender, with clear mucus noted at the os. A cervix that is blue-tinged (cyanotic in appearance) indicates possible pregnancy. A nulliparous os is oval or round; a parous os is slit-like (Figure 4.3). Abnormalities may include the presence of redness, friability, tenderness, lesions, and abnormal cervical mucus.

FAST FACTS in a NUTSHELL

If a visible lesion is noted on the cervix, a colposcopy is recommended regardless of the Pap smear result. This is important even and especially if the Pap smear report is negative.

COLLECTING THE CERVICAL PAP SMEAR (AND OPTIONAL STI TESTING)

Sample the ectocervix, or outer cervix (visible to you during the speculum exam), with either a cervical sampling broom or a plastic spatula. Carry out sampling in a smooth, continuous manner (without disconnecting from the cervix), circling the cervix once when using the spatula and three to five times when using a broom (Figure 4.4). The broom samples both the ectocervix and the endocervix simultaneously so only one collection tool is needed when this device is used.

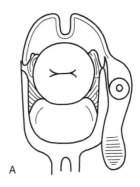

FIGURE 4.3 Inspecting the cervix.
(A) Multiparous cervix.
(B) Nulliparous cervix.

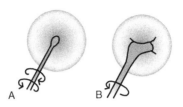

FIGURE 4.4 Pap smear collection technique.

(A) Procedure for collecting endocervical sample for Pap smear and culture for gonorrhea and chlamydia testing using a cotton swab or cytobrush: insert the cotton swab or cytobrush into the os and rotate 360 degrees clockwise. Vigorously mix sample in vial of liquid.

(B) Procedure for collecting ectocervical sample for Pap smear: firmly place the longer projection of the notched end of the Ayre spatula into the os and rotate 360 degrees; hold the horizontal surface containing the sample in the upright position as you withdraw the spatula. Place the flat side of the spatula against the labeled glass slide and smear uniformly across the slide, using one firm motion.

FAST FACTS in a NUTSHELL

"Do it yourself Pap." With the cytobrush in position at the cervical os, ask the patient to cough. This causes the cervix to descend, resulting in the cervix "taking its own Pap smear" while you simply rotate the cytobrush.

Place the sampling tools in the liquid-filled vial, rubbing the collection tools together, mixing vigorously. Next, remove the spatula and cytobrush collection tools from the vial and discard. When using the broom, swirl it vigorously in the vial, and then snap the broom tip off into the collection vial.

With the availability of various new commercial poly- merase chain reaction (PCR), Pap/HPV/STI/vaginitis testing systems (Genpath, MDL, Quest, and others) it is now possible to collect one cervical or one cervicovaginal or lesion sample and obtain samples for multiple screening tests from this one collection. These new testing systems are quick, easy, accu- rate, and affordable and provide a new, improved approach to testing in the context of the gynecologic exam.

OTHER DIAGNOSTIC TESTS TO CONSIDER PERFORMING DURING THE SPECULUM EXAM

Conducting vaginal pH and amine/KOH/whiff testing and vaginal microscopy/wet mount/hanging drop should be considered if indicated based on history, risk factors, and exam findings. Exam findings that suggest further test- ing include abnormal vaginal discharge and/or the pres- ence of lesions, rashes, or tenderness. The process of performing and documenting these tests is summarized in Appendices B and C.

The vaginal sample should carefully be obtained from the **lateral** vaginal wall using a plastic spatula (preferred) or a Dacron swab. Use care to avoid introducing cervical samples, as this mucus is more alkaline and can interfere with accu- rate vaginal pH testing. If vaginal pH or amine/KOH test results are abnormal, vaginal microscopy and/or STI vagini- tis lab testing (PCR or non-PCR) should be considered. The differential diagnosis of vaginal infections is summarized in Table 4.2.

TABLE 4.2 Differential Diagnosis of Vaginal Infections

Condition	Vulvovaginal Symptoms	Vaginal Discharge	Lactobacilli	pH	Microscopy
Candida sp., yeast	Mild to severe itching and vulvovaginal erythema	Variable quality/quantity Classic: white, clumpy "curd-like"	Variable	<4.7	KOH or saline Hyphae, pseudohyphae, and/or spores "Spaghetti and meatballs"
Bacterial vaginosis	Variable; itching absent to mild Mild irritation Possible mild vulvovaginal erythema	Coaty, white, malodorous discharge Fishy odor, particularly after intercourse and with menses	Few	>4.6	Saline Clue cells Few WBCs, KOH/amine test positive
Trichomonas	Variable; mild to severe vulvar itching Petechiae of cervix "strawberry cervix", vulvar erythema, ulceration	Variable quality/quantity, Yellow-green May be frothy Malodorous	Variable	>4.6	Saline Trichomonads Many WBCs KOH/amine test +/–
Atrophic vaginitis	Pruritus, irritation Vulvovaginal dryness and dyspareunia Smooth vaginal walls Few lactobacilli	Red, tender vulva and vagina Variable discharge, lack of rugae Few lactobacilli	Few	>4.6	Saline Parabasal cells WBCs variable, KOH/amine test negative
Desquamative inflammatory vaginitis	Erythema; diffuse or focal of vulva and vagina Pruritus, irritation Dyspareunia	Variable; yellow-green, may be copious No odor	Few	>4.6	Saline Many parabasal, basal cells Many WBCs, KOH/amine test negative Few lactobacilli

53

REMOVING THE SPECULUM

To loosen the speculum's "grip" on the cervix, open the speculum blades slightly as you back the speculum away from the cervix. This is especially important when removing a Welch Allyn speculum, which can be challenging to release from the cervix.

Once the speculum is free of the cervix, close the speculum blades and remove the speculum. Apply slight downward pressure to avoid traumatizing the clitoral area. On occasion, a non-Welch Allyn plastic speculum can be difficult to unlock. Unlocking the blades is required to close the speculum, allowing easy and painless removal.

=====*FAST FACTS in a NUTSHELL*

If you are unable to unlock and release the plastic speculum blades, try not to panic! Take a deep breath, ask the patient to cough forcefully, and quickly remove the open speculum. Try to avoid traumatizing the clitoral area as you remove the speculum.

DISCARDING THE SPECULUM

Plastic specula are single use and should be properly discarded, and metal specula are sterilized/autoclaved and reused. Do not discard the speculum immediately as you may need to obtain additional vaginal samples for vaginal pH, amine/KOH testing, vaginal microscopy, or STI vaginitis testing (Figure 4.5).

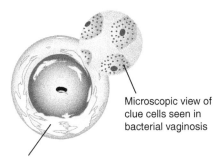

Microscopic view of clue cells seen in bacterial vaginosis

A. View of cervix through speculum

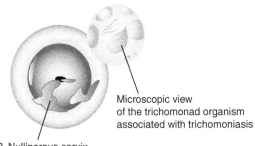

Microscopic view of the trichomonad organism associated with trichomoniasis

B. Nulliparous cervix

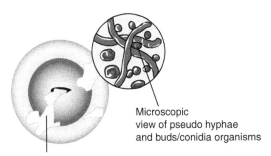

Microscopic view of pseudo hyphae and buds/conidia organisms

C. Multiparous cervix

FIGURE 4.5

(**A**) View of cervix through speculum.
(**B**) Nulliparous cervix.
(**C**) Multiparous cervix.

SAMPLE DOCUMENTATION OF THE VULVAR AND SPECULUM PORTION OF THE GYNECOLOGIC EXAM

External genitalia: Normal distribution of pubic hair and normal anatomy. No masses, lesions, abnormal discharge, tenderness, or good muscle tone

Vagina: Pink; rugated without bulging or lesions; scant opaque white discharge without odor. Vaginal pH 4.0 (normal), amine/KOH test negative, vaginal microscopy negative for clue cells, trichomonads, yeast forms, or white blood cells (WBCs)

Cervix: Pink, smooth, no lesions or mucopus; nontender no cervical motion tenderness (CMT)

5

The Bimanual Exam

INTRODUCTION

*The bimanual exam allows you to assess the patient's
vagina, cervix, uterus, and ovaries. It should be performed in a gentle but thorough manner, first palpating
the vagina, then the uterus, ovaries, and, if indicated,
the rectovaginal structures and rectum last.*

In this chapter you will learn how to:

1. Perform the bimanual examination for palpating the uterus and ovaries.
2. Perform a rectovaginal exam.

The traditional approach is to perform the speculum exam
prior to conducting the bimanual exam. However, some clinicians recommend conducting the bimanual exam prior to
the speculum exam. Advantages to this sequence include less
patient discomfort with the speculum exam, an opportunity
to locate the cervix prior to speculum insertion, and less need
for lubrication with the speculum exam.

==*FAST FACTS in a NUTSHELL*

In women of reproductive age, you may not be able to palpate the ovaries during the bimanual examination. This is not cause for alarm nor does it require additional testing unless the patient is symptomatic or high risk for ovarian cancer, or unless you suspect other conditions such as endometriosis. In contrast, if you palpate ovaries in a menopausal patient, consider this abnormal, and conduct a thorough work-up to rule out pathology.

THE BIMANUAL EXAM

The bimanual exam is conducted while standing at the foot of the examination table with the patient's buttocks at the end of the table. Place one gloved hand on the lower abdomen just above the mid-suprapubic area and, using a small amount of lubricant, insert one, or preferably two, gloved fingers into the vagina. Using the lubricant reduces patient discomfort and facilitates the exam. Begin the bimanual exam by thoroughly palpating the vagina and cervix, noting areas of tenderness or masses.

To palpate the uterus, gently apply suprapubic pressure, while positioning your fingertips under the cervix and gently lift up. Assess the uterus for position (angle), size, shape, contour, mobility, and tenderness. Note any abnormal findings such as tenderness (suggesting pelvic inflammatory disease [PID]), masses (suggesting fibroids), and lack of mobility (possible endometriosis).

The position of the uterus within the pelvis varies. See Figure 5.1, Positions of the uterus. An anteverted uterus is angled toward the abdomen while a retroverted uterus is angled toward the tailbone and rectum. Bimanual palpation of the anteverted uterus is shown in Figure 5.2.

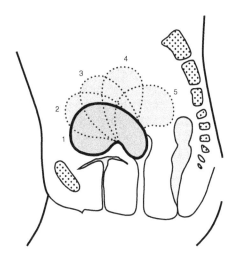

FIGURE 5.1 Positions of the uterus. (1) Anteflexed, (2) anteverted, (3) midposition, (4) retroverted, and (5) retroflexed (from Carcio, H. A., & Secor, M. C. [2010]. *Advanced health assessment of women: Clinical skills and procedures* [2nd ed., p. 9]. New York, NY: Springer Publishing Company.)

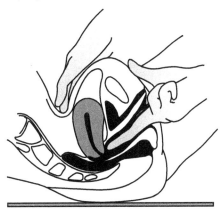

FIGURE 5.2 Bimanual palpation of the anteverted uterus (from Carcio, H. A., & Secor, M. C. [2010]. *Advanced health assessment of women: Clinical skills and procedures* [2nd ed., p. 75]. New York, NY: Springer Publishing Company.)

A normal uterus is approximately the size of a lemon or small pear but can range in size somewhat. The uterus is normally smooth, semifirm, nontender, and mobile. If the uterus is tender, rule out PID. If the uterus is diffusely enlarged, rule out pregnancy and consider additional diagnostic testing based on the history, exam, and differential diagnosis. If the uterus is irregular and unusually firm, suspect fibroids and confirm with transvaginal ultrasound and/or hysteroscopy. See Figure 5.3, Appearance of uterine fibroids.

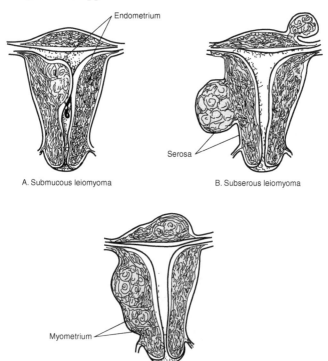

A. Submucous leiomyoma

B. Subserous leiomyoma

C. Intramural leiomyoma

FIGURE 5.3 Appearance of uterine fibroids (from Carcio, H. A., & Secor, M. C. [2010]. *Advanced health assessment of women: Clinical skills and procedures* [2nd ed., p. 77]. New York, NY: Springer Publishing Company.)

The uterus is not always easy to palpate, especially if the patient is obese, anxious, physically disabled, or elderly. Examining these special populations is discussed in Chapter 10.

FAST FACTS in a NUTSHELL

If the uterus is not palpable suprapubically, it may be retroverted, or "tipped" back toward the patient's tailbone. In this case, the uterus may be palpable only by rectovaginal exam (Figure 5.4).

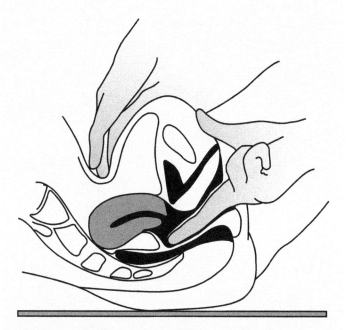

FIGURE 5.4 Bimanual palpation of the retroverted uterus (from Carcio, H. A., & Secor, M. C. [2010]. *Advanced health assessment of women: Clinical skills and procedures* [2nd ed., p. 76]. New York, NY: Springer Publishing Company.)

THE ADNEXAL EXAM

Perform the adnexal exam next. During this part of the exam, you'll examine the ovaries, which are located lateral to the fundus of the uterus and are about the size of almonds. Assess the ovaries for size (enlarged), shape (masses), and tenderness.

To examine the ovaries (Figure 5.5):

1. Move your abdominal hand to either the right or left lateral lower abdomen area, just lateral to the fundus of the uterus.
2. Position the fingers of the vaginal hand in the vaginal fornix of the adnexal side being examined.
3. Apply pressure similar to that you use to palpate the uterus.
4. Repeat this same technique on the opposite side to examine the second ovary.

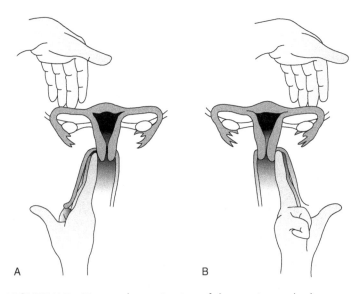

A   B

FIGURE 5.5 Bimanual examination of the ovaries and adenexae. From Carcio, H. A. (1998). *Management of the infertile woman* (p. 100). Philadelphia: Lippincott. Adapted from Gray, R. H. (1980). *Manual for the provision of intrauterine devices* (p. 98). Geneva, Switzerland: World Health Organization.

Ovaries normally are almond sized, nontender, and semifirm (Table 5.1); however, not uncommonly, they may not be palpable. Endometriosis may cause the ovaries to be located behind the uterus (referred to as "holding hands"), and so they will not be palpable. Cystic enlargement of the ovaries will feel like fullness in the affected adnexal area and may be tender or nontender. A tubal pregnancy is indistinguishable clinically from an ovarian cyst, so additional testing is urgently needed to determine the underlying etiology. This may include pelvic ultrasound, pregnancy testing, CBC with differential, CA125, and a sedimentation rate. A history of unprotected intercourse and late menses increases the risk of pregnancy and the clinician's index of suspicion.

The ovaries may be palpable without conducting a rectovaginal exam, but when they are not palpable on the vaginal bimanual exam, the rectovaginal bimanual exam may be particularly helpful (see Chapter 6).

The fallopian tubes, considered part of the adnexae (Exhibit 5.1), are not typically palpable, due to their small size. They are approximately 5 inches in length, about half the diameter of a pencil, and rubbery. If palpable, consider the possibility of salpingitis or endometriosis.

TABLE 5.1 Assessment Findings of the Uterus and Adnexae: Normal and Abnormal

Findings of Area Assessed	
Normal	**Abnormal**
Uterus	
Approximate size of a lemon	Enlargement = may indicate pregnancy or other mass
Normally smooth, semifirm, nontender, and mobile	Tender = possible PID or endometriosis Irregular = may suggest fibroids
Position Most often, anteverted, anteflexed (angled toward the abdomen) Freely movable	Retroverted, retroflexed (angled toward the tailbone) uterus may be difficult to palpate bimanually; a rectovaginal exam may be required. May be result of endometriosis

(continued)

TABLE 5.1 *(continued)*

Findings of Area Assessed

Normal	Abnormal
Adnexae	
Ovaries Size: almond size Nontender, semifirm, and mobile	Enlargement: may be due to cystic enlargement, polycystic ovarian syndrome (PCOS), or tubal pregnancy; palpation will convey sense of "fullness"; may be tender. Further testing is required to distinguish Endometriosis: may push ovaries to relocate behind the uterus, position is called "holding hands"
Postmenopausal—usually not palpable	If palpable, consider abnormal and investigate
Fallopian tubes Normal: about 5 inches in length, rubbery, half-diameter of a pencil, not palpable, and nontender	If palpable, consider salpingitis or an ectopic pregnancy If palpable and feel like fibrous bands, consider previous salpingitis or endometriosis

Adapted from Carcio, H. A., & Secor, M. C. (2010). *Advanced health assessment of women: Clinical skills and procedures* (2nd ed., pp. 5–6, 78–79, 529). New York, NY: Springer Publishing Company; and Rhoads, J. (2006). *Advanced health assessment and diagnostic reasoning* (p. 341). Philadelphia, PA: Lippincott Williams & Wilkins.

Exhibit 5.1 Sample Documentation of the Vulvar, Speculum, and Bimanual Portions of the Gynecologic Exam

External genitalia: Normal distribution of pubic hair and normal anatomy. No masses, lesions, abnormal discharge, or tenderness.

(continued)

Exhibit 5.1 *(continued)*

Vagina: Pink; rugated without bulging or lesions; scant opaque white discharge without odor; good muscle tone. Vaginal pH 4.0 (normal), amine/KOH test negative, vaginal microscopy negative for clue cells, trichomonads, yeast forms, or WBCs.

Cervix: Pink, smooth, no lesions or mucopus; nontender, no cervical motion tenderness (CMT).

Uterus: Anteverted, normal size, shape, contour (NSSC), mobile, nontender, without palpable masses.

Adnexae: Ovaries palpated, normal size, nontender, and no masses palpated.

Rectovaginal: No lesions, masses, or fissures; nontender, small amount of brown soft stool present, guaiac test negative.

6

The Rectal Exam

INTRODUCTION

Increasing awareness of anorectal cancer risk and associated risk factors requires heightened vigilance when conducting the rectal exam. Approximately 90% of anal cancers are associated with high-risk human papillomavirus (HR-HPV) infection. Risk factors and risk populations for anal dysplasia include HIV infection; men who have sex with men (MSM); certain immunocompromised conditions, such as transplant patients; history of HPV infection, including anal and/or perineal condyloma; and a history of significant abnormal Pap smears, such as moderate to severe dysplasia, including cervical intraepithelial neoplasia (CIN) 2 and 3.

In this chapter you will learn:

1. The indications for performing a rectal exam.
2. The technique for performing a rectal examination.
3. The risk factors and high-risk populations for anal dysplasia.
4. The technique for performing an anal Pap smear.
5. How to perform a guaiac stool test for occult blood.

THE RECTOVAGINAL EXAM

Considerations for performing a rectovaginal exam include the patient's age (especially older than 50 years), risk factors, and need to more fully assess the uterus, ovaries, rectovaginal septum, and rectum. The rectovaginal exam is particularly helpful if the uterus is retroverted and/or if the ovaries are not palpable vaginally. Other indications include gastrointestinal (GI) complaints, risk factors such as a history of reproductive or GI cancers, an unsatisfactory vaginal bimanual exam, obesity, or when other pathology such as an ovarian mass is suspected.

INDICATIONS

The rectal exam may be part of a thorough bimanual exam and should be conducted based on the patient's age, risk factors, medical history, and health status. Generally, a rectal exam is recommended for:

- Women over 50 years of age
- Younger women based on risk factors and clinical indications

=====*FAST FACTS in a NUTSHELL*

In certain patients, particularly those with a retroverted uterus, obesity, or risks for reproductive cancers such as ovarian or uterine cancer, the rectal exam may enhance palpating the uterus and ovaries.

The rectal exam may be embarrassing and slightly uncomfortable for the patient, but can provide valuable clinical information. It must be performed gently and thoroughly while providing education and emotional support to the patient throughout the exam.

The patient may be positioned in a supine, lithotomy position utilizing gynecologic stirrups or in a side lying position with one or both knees slightly bent.

EXTERNAL RECTAL EXAM

Begin the rectal exam by visually inspecting the external rectal area, using care in separating and inspecting the skin folds that comprise the external sphincter. Note abnormalities including erythema, whitening, swelling, tenderness, and masses, and other lesions such as fissures, blisters, and ulcers. Next, palpate these tissues and any masses for tenderness, and other abnormal findings.

RECTOVAGINAL EXAM

To prepare for the exam, change your gloves and use sufficient lubricant to facilitate the exam and minimize patient discomfort. Insert your index finger vaginally and your middle finger rectally. Ask the patient to "bear down, relax, and then slowly inhale and exhale." Slide your fingers into place as the patient is "bearing down" and exhaling. This exam is considered invasive and somewhat uncomfortable (Carcio & Secor, 2010, pp. 78–79).

- Palpate the rectovaginal septum.
- With your other hand on the abdomen, push the uterus as posteriorly as possible.
- With the internal fingers, assess the posterior surface of the uterus and the rectal wall to assess the rectal walls, the rectovaginal septum, and the cul-de-sac for tenderness or masses.

- Note any masses, tenderness, hemorrhoids, or the presence of a retroverted uterus.
- If the uterus is retroverted or retroflexed, the fundus may not be palpable. If palpable, note characteristics such as size, contour, firmness, tenderness, masses, and mobility.
  - If the uterus is retroverted due to endometriosis, it may be fixed and nonmobile.
  - Endometriosis may be further evaluated by assessing nodularity of the uterosacral ligaments.

INTERNAL RECTAL EXAM

Perform the internal exam wearing new gloves and using adequate lubrication to facilitate the exam and provide maximum comfort to the patient.

Gently insert one gloved finger and check for unusual tenderness, masses, and any other abnormal findings (Table 6.1). Note the presence, consistency, and color of any stool, and perform a guaiac test to check for occult blood.

Procedure for Guaiac Test

- Upon removal from the rectum, test a guaiac stool sample for occult blood by rolling your third gloved finger onto the test card, when indicated.
- Apply three drops of developing solution to the opposite side of the card.
- The test is positive if you note any blue color.

The guaiac test is most accurate when patients perform the test at home after following special dietary restrictions. The patient collects three stool samples on separate days and returns the samples to the office or lab for guaiac testing.

========================*FAST FACTS in a NUTSHELL*

Colonoscopy is the gold standard test for identifying gastrointestinal pathology such as polyps and precancerous and cancerous lesions.

ANAL CYTOLOGY

With the risk of anal dysplasia on the rise, increasingly, clinicians are performing anal Pap smears in certain high-risk patients. Risk factors, high-risk populations for anal dysplasia, and the recommended procedure for performing an anal Pap smear are reviewed in Exhibit 6.1.

Exhibit 6.1 Procedure for Performing an Anal Pap Smear

Indications

There are no national recommendations, but the following high-risk patients may be considered for anal dysplasia/carcinoma screening:

- Current candidates: MSM or HIV-infected persons
- Possible candidates: Those who are immunocompromised; those with HPV-related disease, especially vulvar intraepithelial neoplasia (VIN); and men and women with perianal genital warts, or human papilloma virus (HPV)

(*continued*)

Exhibit 6.1 (*continued*)

- Other possible candidates and risk factors: Those who have had 15 or more sexual partners, unprotected receptive anal intercourse, a history of cervical intraepithelial neoplasia (CIN), or cigarette smokers

Procedure

- Patient should avoid anal intercourse and douching 24 hours before test.
- Set up supplies and equipment in advance.
- Educate patient about procedure and rationale for the test.
- Position patient side lying (left side) or lithotomy using gynecologic stirrups.
- Drape patient.
- Moisten a Dacron swab with tap water.
  - Avoid using a cytobrush because it may cause patient discomfort.
- Insert swab approximately 5 cm (2 inches) until the swab reaches the rectal vault.
  - A slight decrease in resistance can be felt.
  - If significant resistance is encountered, remove the swab and redirect the angle or position of the swab.
- Rotate swab 360 degrees.
  - Use a spiral motion and firm pressure against the lateral walls of the anal canal.
  - Circle in one direction only, as reversing direction may remove sample that has been collected.

(continued)

- Gradually withdraw over 10 seconds, while still rotating.
- Agitate sample in liquid fixative for 10 to 15 seconds.
- Label sample as "Anal source."

Interpretation of Results

- Anal Pap smears are interpreted using similar nomenclature and classifications as cervical Pap smears: negative for malignancy, ASC-US, ASC-H, LSIL, HSIL
- No reflex HPV testing is available currently.
- Anal abnormalities are referred for high resolution anoscopy (HRA) and possible biopsy.

TABLE 6.1 Assessment Findings of the Rectum and Anus: Normal and Abnormal

Normal	Abnormal
Rectovaginal: areas examined should be smooth, firm, nonfriable, and nontender	Polyps Lesions Hemorrhoids Bleeding following palpation
Palpation of uterus: uncomfortable, but not painful	Pain: suggests endometriosis or PID

FAST FACTS in a NUTSHELL

Sample Documentation of a Complete Gynecologic Exam with Normal Findings

External genitalia: Normal distribution of pubic hair and normal anatomy. No masses, lesions, abnormal discharge, or tenderness

Vagina: Pink; rugated without bulging or lesions; scant opaque white discharge without odor; good muscle tone. Vaginal pH 4.0 (normal), amine/KOH test negative, vaginal microscopy negative for clue cells, trichomonads, yeast forms, or WBCs

Cervix: Pink, smooth, no lesions or mucopus; nontender, no cervical motion tenderness (CMT)

Uterus: Anteverted; normal size, shape, contour (NSSC); mobile; nontender; without palpable masses

Adnexae: Ovaries palpated, normal size, nontender, and no masses palpated

Rectovaginal: No lesions, masses, or fissures; nontender; small amount of brown, soft stool present; guaiac test negative

Approach to Examining Special Populations

Many factors can contribute to challenging pelvic exams. Some challenges occur with menopause as part of the normal aging process and others are related to very specific events such as previous assault and trauma. Depending on age, body type, and childbirth history normal pelvic landmarks may shift and certain pelvic structures can be difficult to locate. In this section of the book we provide practical suggestions for the resolution of some of the more common difficulties you may encounter in practice.

7

Specific "Challenges"

INTRODUCTION

The ability to adequately visualize both the external and internal genitalia is foundational to performing a complete pelvic exam. Many factors can interfere with your ability to see and examine pelvic organs. This chapter will review important steps that can help you "find" the cervix in challenging clinical situations and improve comfort for patients who are experiencing pain and vulvar itching.

In this chapter you will learn:

1. Common reasons for difficulty visualizing the cervix.
2. Recommended strategies for improving visualization.
3. Tips for increasing comfort during the pelvic exam in patients with vulvar pain and itching.

DIFFICULT VISUALIZATION OF CERVIX

Proper visualization of the cervix is important for an adequate Pap smear sample. Even if you are not performing Pap smear testing, you should inspect the cervix for abnormalities such as inflammation, discharge, bleeding, and lesions. The cervix often comes into view when the speculum has been inserted and opened. Occasionally, the cervix may be difficult to view and requires you to use different techniques.

A cervix that is not positioned in the midline is a common reason for difficult visualization. If you cannot see the cervix easily, you should withdraw the speculum and manually palpate the cervix to determine the location. When you reinsert the speculum, angle it toward the area where you palpated the cervix. Moving the speculum from side to side slightly and opening it wider may help the cervix come into view.

In addition to repositioning the speculum, having the patient change positions may be helpful. Instruct the patient to move as close to the edge of the table as possible and have her tilt up her hips and buttocks. If she is unable to tilt up her hips enough, placing a small rolled towel under her hips or buttocks may be helpful. Asking her to bear down or cough forcefully may also bring the cervix into view.

It is also difficult to visualize a cervix that is located in an extreme posterior position. Palpating will reveal the posterior location. A standard, disposable plastic speculum will often not provide adequate visualization of a cervix in this position. It is often necessary to use a large, extra long speculum to complete the exam. Having the patient bear down, flex her hips upward, and retract her knees closer to her body will help move the cervix down and forward.

Another reason for not locating the cervix is that the woman has relaxed or weakened vaginal walls that impede visualization. In these situations, excess loose tissue on the side walls of the vagina collapses inward and blocks the opening of the speculum. One solution is to try the largest speculum available and open it as wide as possible in order to keep the lateral walls apart. Another solution is to cut the finger off a glove (or use a condom and remove the tip to form an improvised sheath). Placing this over the speculum blades will help hold back the vaginal walls once the speculum is opened. A lateral-wall retractor can also be used but is often not commonly available in outpatient settings.

―――――――――――――*FAST FACTS in a NUTSHELL*

Documentation
- It is important to document any variations on normal position of pelvic organs. Examples:
  - "Cervix is posterior, deviated to the patient's right."
  - "Cervix difficult to visualize due to redundant vaginal wall tissue."

Communication

When pelvic exams take extra time or manipulation of equipment and positions, it is not uncommon for patients to feel as if there is something wrong with their anatomy that is making it difficult for you to complete the exam. Reassurance should be given that the cervix, uterus, and ovaries can be in different positions, and this does not necessarily indicate an abnormality. Pregnancy, childbirth, a large weight gain or loss, and menopause can all cause a slight shift in pelvic organs. To decrease any anxiety, it is essential to let the patient know what you are doing and why. Statements such as "I need to move the speculum so I can see your cervix clearly" keep the patient informed about the exam without suggesting that their body is abnormal.

Follow-Up

With the use of different techniques, it is often possible to visualize a cervix that is initially difficult to see. If it is still impossible to clearly see the cervix, the practitioner can attempt a blind sweep of the cervix to obtain a Pap smear specimen, and if gonorrhea or chlamydia cultures are indicated, they can be sent with a urine sample and/or a vaginal sample. If necessary, the patient can be rescheduled for a follow-up visit at a different time and the pelvic exam reattempted.

FAST FACTS in a NUTSHELL

Repositioning the patient and the speculum may bring the cervix into view.

VULVAR AND VAGINAL PAIN

Patients who experience pain of the vulvar and vaginal area often have difficulty tolerating the pelvic exam, and clinicians who treat these patients need to conduct the exam slowly and gently. Pain can result from trauma or injury to the area, infections, skin conditions such as lichen sclerosis or psoriasis, and thin, dry skin that can occur with menopause. Vulvar pain can also result from vulvodynia. This condition causes pain, burning, and/or irritation of the vulvar. There is no definitive test for vulvodynia and it is often a diagnosis of exclusion based on the patient's symptoms, presence of allodynia, and lack of any identifiable cause of the pain.

Regardless of the cause, performing a pelvic exam on a woman with vulvar and/or vaginal pain can be extremely challenging. Using a small or pediatric speculum may help decrease discomfort and allow you to visualize the cervix. If even the smallest speculum causes too much pain, Pap smear collection can be attempted without visualizing the cervix, although it is unlikely that this will result in a sample that includes endocervical cells. Vaginal samples for wet mount examination can be gathered with a small swab, and testing for gonorrhea and chlamydia can be done with a urine or vaginal sample (see Appendices B and C).

FAST FACTS in a NUTSHELL

Documentation

- For patients with a complaint of vulvar and vaginal pain, it is important to document the location and quality of pain. Examples:
  - "Tenderness and allodynia bilaterally with gentle palpation with a cotton swab."
  - "Vaginal atrophy and dryness (positive sticky glove test) present from 5 to 7 o'clock at the introitus; able to complete exam with narrow speculum."

Communication

Pain is subjective and therefore the patient will be the best source of information. It is important to determine the onset, duration, location, and quality. Also, you should assess any treatments that have been tried and whether they were successful. Patients with chronic pain who do not have any outward symptoms often feel as if no one believes their discomfort is real, especially if they have seen many providers for the same issue. It is important to let patients know that you understand their discomfort is real, even if you cannot immediately identify a cause.

Follow-Up

Follow-up appointments can be scheduled as needed based on exam findings. If a diagnosis can be established and treatment started, a return visit can be scheduled to assess response to treatment. Infections, skin conditions, and atrophy can be treated and the exam deferred until healing has taken place.

VULVAR AND VAGINAL ITCHING

Significant vulvar and vaginal itching can also cause considerable discomfort. Vulvitis can be caused by allergic and contact reactions, inflammatory responses, dermatological conditions, and fungal, viral, and bacterial infections. It is a common gynecological complaint and results in approximately 17 million office visits each year. Inflammation associated with the underlying cause of the itching makes the skin fragile, and often patients with vulvar itching will have excoriated skin from scratching and inflammation. It is not uncommon to see fissuring and cracking of the genital skin, especially if the itching and/or condition is chronic. See Table 7.1, Common Causes of Vulvar Itching and Associated Treatment.

TABLE 7.1 Common Causes of Vulvar Itching and Associated Treatment

Possible Causes	Treatment
Fungal infections (yeast)	Topical and oral antifungal medications
Bacterial infections (BV)	Oral and topical antibiotics
Sexually transmitted infections	Antibiotics or antivirals specific to the infection
Allergic reactions and/or Contact dermatitis	Removal of allergen; topical or oral steroids; antihistamines; sitz baths, improved hygiene, emollients
Skin conditions (lichen simplex chronicus, lichen sclerosus, lichen planus, psoriasis)	Topical steroids, improved hygiene, emollients
Atrophic vaginitis	Local estrogen, improved hygiene, emollients

Inspection of the genital skin will show the extent of erythema, irritation, or excoriation associated with inflammation and itching. Skin is often tender and sensitive to touch. Clinicians should be gentle and take care to not injure the skin further during the exam. If the condition is acute and the patient is due for a routine exam with Pap smear, it may be advisable to treat the immediate problem and reschedule the routine exam after healing has occurred. Swabs for wet mount examination can be taken without the use of a speculum, and testing for gonorrhea and chlamydia can be done with a urine or vaginal sample.

FAST FACTS in a NUTSHELL

Documentation
- Areas of redness or excoriation should be documented clearly. Examples:
  - "Erythema and fissuring of vulvar bilaterally."
  - "Erythema of vaginal walls and introitus especially between 5 and 7 o'clock."
- Any vaginal discharge needs to be noted. Examples:
  - "Moderate thin, white discharge coating vaginal walls."
  - "Thick, clumpy white discharge present."

Communication

In all cases of vulvar and vaginal itching, an in-office wet prep (wet mount, vaginal microscopy) should be performed to assess for yeast, bacterial vaginosis (BV), trichomoniasis (see Chapter 3), and atrophic vaginitis. Results of the wet prep can be communicated immediately and a treatment plan promptly initiated. Discussions with patients need to include education regarding the type of infection and course of treatment. All women with complaints of vulvar and vaginal itching should be discouraged from douching or using strong or drying soaps, scented vaginal hygiene products, and tight and restrictive pants and undergarments, especially thong underwear, and shaving pubic hair.

Follow-Up

As with pain, follow-up for vulvar itching will be determined primarily by the diagnosis and choice of treatment. Uncomplicated fungal infections usually respond well to antifungal medications and often clear quickly with treatment. Inflammatory allergic reactions resolve with removal of the allergen. Skin that is extremely excoriated should be reevaluated for healing and monitored for the development of a secondary bacterial infection. A full exam can be deferred until healing is under way and the patient is more comfortable.

FAST FACTS in a NUTSHELL

- For patients with pain, use the smallest speculum size possible.
- You can gather specimens with a small swab or urine if the patient is unable to tolerate a speculum exam.

For further information related to specific pelvic exam challenges and potential resolutions, please see Appendix A.

8

Examining the Patient With Anxiety, History of Sexual Abuse, or Vaginismus

INTRODUCTION

Many women are anxious during gynecologic exams, but some women are extremely anxious. Sometimes a cause for the anxiety cannot be determined, but extreme anxiety can also be associated with specific events, such as a history of sexual abuse. Vaginismus, or abnormal involuntary spasms of the vagina, can be a result of sexual abuse or trauma and causes increased pain and inability to tolerate a gynecologic exam. During the interviewing process, a thorough psychological, social, family, and sexual history should be obtained, noting evidence of or past history of anxiety, sexual abuse, family trauma, negative gynecologic experiences, and other factors that might indicate the patient may have difficulty with gynecologic exams.

In this chapter you will learn how to:

1. Recognize behaviors that signal extreme anxiety and apply strategies to help the patient work through the pelvic exam.
2. Approach a pelvic exam with a patient who has a history of sexual abuse.
3. Use techniques for completing a pelvic exam on a patient who has vaginismus.

ANXIETY

A severely anxious patient can be very challenging to examine and make completing a pelvic exam difficult. If the patient has previously had a gynecologic exam, she should be asked about prior experiences and any difficulties she had. Women who are having their first exam should be told exactly what to expect. They may benefit from seeing the speculum, and some women may want to hold it and try opening and closing it.

Women who are extremely anxious should be talked through the entire exam. This will allow them to know exactly what is happening and in what order the exam will proceed. Women should know they can ask you to stop the exam at any time and you will honor their request. Proceed with the exam slowly and gently. Communicate in a relaxed and unhurried manner. If the patient is known to the practice and previous exams have been difficult, allow extra time.

Encourage relaxation techniques, including deep breathing, meditation, and imagery. The patient may benefit from a support person of her choice, and, if possible, should be allowed to have her support present with her for the exam. If speculum insertion is difficult, consider asking the patient to bear down and breathe deeply. It may take multiple attempts to insert the speculum and complete the exam *occurring over multiple visits and sometimes many months.* Palpating the cervix in advance of the speculum exam may help both the patient and the clinician.

Consider short-acting antianxiety medications if the patient has a support person who is able to drive her home after the exam. The decision to prescribe antianxiety medications should be based on the patient's clinical history, current medications, and preferences. Caution should be used in patients with a history of substance abuse. All antianxiety medications have side effects of drowsiness and dizziness and patients should be informed of this. See Table 8.1 for common antianxiety medications and available doses. It is often helpful to have patients take the prescribed dose 30 minutes prior to their exam.

TABLE 8.1 Short-Acting Antianxiety Medications (Benzodiazepines)*

Medication (Generic, Brand Name)	Single dose (mg) prior to exam
Lorazapam (Ativan)	0.5, 1, or 2
Alprazolam (Xanax)	0.25, 0.5, 1, or 2
Clonazepam (Klonopin)	0.5, 1, or 2
Diazepam (Valium)	2, 5, or 10

*These medications should be used with caution, especially with women who have a history of addiction or mental health issues.

FAST FACTS in a NUTSHELL

Documentation

- Physiologic signs of anxiety should be documented. Examples:
  - "Tachycardic, HR 94."
  - "Patient diaphoretic, tense, and guarding."
- Extent to which the exam can be completed is documented. Examples:
  - "Exam performed; bimanual limited by *patient* anxiety, *unable to accurately assess uterus and ovaries.*"
  - "Unable to insert speculum or perform bimanual exam *due to anxiety and/or pain when exam attempted.*"

Communication

Patients with extreme anxiety are often upset over the difficulties with the exam and apologetic that the process is longer or incomplete. Providers should remain patient, calm, and understanding. Provider anxiety or frustration will only increase the patient's anxiety. Each aspect of the exam should be done slowly, at a pace that is set by the patient. It is important for the provider to communicate during each step. This will allow the patient to decide if she is able to continue. At the completion of the exam, the woman should be informed of all findings and if any follow-up is needed.

Follow-Up

If the exam can be completed *and is normal,* then follow-up is not necessary. If anxiety prevents all or part of the exam, then a plan should be made for repeating the exam at a different time. If this is necessary, strategies can be implemented to address the patient's anxiety and therefore increase the likelihood the next exam will be successful. If anxiety is extreme, referral to a therapist may help the patient work through underlying issues related to the gynecologic exam. Bringing a friend and implementing meditation, biofeedback, and other relaxation techniques can also be very effective in reducing anxiety. If anxiety is not specific to the gynecologic exam and part of an overall anxiety disorder, referral to a mental health provider should be considered to have mental health issues evaluated and treated.

FAST FACTS in a NUTSHELL

- Encourage use of a mirror and patient involvement during the exam process.
- Proceed with the exam slowly and thoroughly, and explain the exam simply (especially in advance) to decrease anxiety.
- Encourage relaxation techniques and deep breathing.
- Consider short-acting antianxiety medications if appropriate for the patient and situation.

SEXUAL ABUSE

Performing a pelvic exam on a patient with a history of sexual abuse can be especially challenging. It is extremely important to not re-victimize the patient during the exam. Exposure and touching of the pelvic area and positioning for the exam often bring up memories of the abuse. Many women who have experienced sexual abuse or assault do not disclose this to their health care provider. Tjaden and Thoennes (2000) reported the 17.6% of women in the National Violence Against Women Survey (NVAWS) were raped at some time in their lives. In the United States, the prevalence of rape is equal to one in every six women (Brown & Muscari, 2010, p. 170). Abuse victims may demonstrate certain behaviors that suggest a history of abuse. During an examination, the woman may be reluctant to undress and allow you access to her pelvic and genital area. The abused woman may also move away as you attempt to insert the speculum or may close her legs tightly. Arching her back off the exam table and having a rigidly tense posture are also actions that are common for abuse victims. Other responses that are possible include crying, shaking, hiding under the drape sheet, or complete disassociation and separation from the exam.

For women with a known abuse history, having control over the flow and timing of the exam is crucial. The visit often takes much longer, and an exam may be impossible or require multiple visits to complete. Abuse victims need to feel secure, and therefore the process from introduction and first visit to the completion of a full exam can take many visits or even years as the patient learns to trust the provider and feel safe. Sexual assault patients should always be greeted and interviewed while fully clothed.

Before beginning any part of the exam, let the patient know exactly what to expect. Some patients feel more comfortable if they have their own support person with them and you should always try to accommodate this request. Being completely undressed is often difficult for sexual abuse victims.

Allowing an abused woman to keep on some clothing, such as her shirt, may increase her comfort.

There are other important steps you can take when performing a gynecologic exam on a woman who has been sexually abused. Letting the patient set the pace of the exam and have control over certain actions can enhance empowerment and increase the chance of a nontraumatic exam. Patients may wish to use a mirror and insert the speculum themselves. The speculum should be warm, the smallest size possible, and inserted slowly. Lubricant should be used to decrease discomfort. Consider alternate positions, such as semireclining and not using stirrups. It is important to assess the patient's anxiety and level of tolerance for the exam multiple times. Let her know that you will stop at any point if she is having difficulty completing the exam.

If it is impossible to complete the exam, the patient may require a step-by-step desensitization process. Over the course of multiple appointments, the patient can become more familiar with the environment and exam process. At this point you might consider co-managing care with a counselor who specializes in sexual abuse.

If the sexual assault or abuse occurred recently, then the genital area should be examined carefully. According to Brown and Muscari (2010, p. 175), many health care providers use the TEARS pneumonic to describe the different types of genital injuries. Becoming familiar with this pneumonic will assist you in identifying the constellation of rape-related injuries experienced by victims of sexual assault:

T = tears, any break in tissue integrity
E = ecchymosis, any discoloration of skin or mucous membranes; also called bruising
A = abrasion, skin excoriations caused by the removal of the most superficial layer of skin
R = redness, erythematous skin that is abnormally inflamed because of irritation
S = swelling, edematous, or transient engorgement of tissues

Brown and Muscari also report the "common genital injuries in elder victims of sexual assault are lacerations, abrasions, and bruises" (2010, p. 185).

Sommers (2007) identifies the most common locations for injury as:

- Posterior fourchette
- Labia minora
- Hymen
- Fossa navicularis

FAST FACTS in a NUTSHELL

Documentation

- With a remote history of sexual assault, documentation includes the woman's emotional response to the exam. Examples:
  - "Mild anxiety verbalized but able to tolerate exam without incident."
  - "Unable to complete exam due to anxiety and emotional distress."

Communication

The timing of the sexual abuse or assault will often guide the discussion before and after the exam. If the abuse has occurred in the past and the patient is stable and out of physical danger, then the conversation will focus on the woman's feelings toward the exam, any previous difficulties she has encountered, and what can be done to increase her comfort with the present exam. If the assault was recent and the woman has not received evaluation and health care since the attack, the conversation will be very different. If the assault has occurred during the past 5 days, the woman should be informed about the collection of forensic evidence (see Follow-Up). If it has been greater than 5 days since the assault, the practitioner should ask about the patient's immediate concerns, such as pregnancy or sexually transmitted infections (STIs).

Follow-Up

A woman's ability to tolerate gynecologic exams after a history of sexual abuse or assault will vary widely. Some women may experience only mild anxiety while others will exhibit symptoms of severe distress. Follow-up plans will be based on the patient's symptoms and feelings about the exam. For those with acute distress that prevents completion of a pelvic exam, follow-up and co-management with a therapist or counselor are often helpful. If the abuse or assault was recent and you are the first provider whom the patient has encountered, information should be provided about rape crisis centers and options regarding reporting to law enforcement. If assaulted within the past 5 to 7 days, the woman should be informed that forensic evidence can be collected. This is best done by a provider who has specialized experience and training in sexual assault exams. You should be aware of what services are available in your practice area if referrals are needed. Additional follow-up for repeat STI or pregnancy testing can also be scheduled based on the timing of the assault.

FAST FACTS in a NUTSHELL

- A successful exam may take months or years to complete.
- Consider co-management with a counselor.
- Use slow, gentle movements and allow the patient direct the pace of the exam.

VAGINISMUS

Vaginismus is an involuntary spasm of the muscles surrounding the vagina. This spasm causes the vagina to become very tight or close completely. Vaginismus can be caused by trauma, such as sexual abuse or assault, or can result from chronic vaginal pain and infection. Vaginismus is often suspected from the patient's history of difficult or impossible vaginal intercourse.

It is important to remember that there are varying degrees of vaginismus. Patients who have a mild form may be able to tolerate a pelvic exam but experience a great amount of discomfort. The most severe forms of vaginismus may make completing a pelvic exam impossible due to a spasm of the vaginal muscles that closes the vagina. For women who experience pain, proceed in much the same way you would for victims of sexual assault: slow movements, small speculum, lubrication, and relaxation techniques. Apply topical lidocaine (5%) either to the patient or to the speculum prior to insertion. If there is a concern about gonorrhea or chlamydia, perform urine or vaginal swab testing. You might also consider performing a limited exam based on what the patient can tolerate. In severe cases of vaginismus, it may be impossible to perform a pelvic exam until the woman has sought treatment. Patience and support are extremely important. As a clinician, you need to understand that performing a complete pelvic exam may take many visits or even years.

FAST FACTS in a NUTSHELL

Documentation

- Documentation should focus on the severity of vaginismus. Examples:
  - "Patient uncomfortable with exam, completed with pediatric speculum."
  - "Unable to insert speculum due to vaginal muscle spasm."

Communication

Patients with vaginismus often complain of difficulty and pain with sexual intercourse. Discussions with patients should include assessment of sexual activity, how vaginismus affects sexual relationships, and any treatments that have been effective in reducing discomfort and spasm. It may take many years before women seek treatment for the disorder due to embarrassment, fear of not being believed, or hoping that the symptoms will resolve on their own. Because vaginismus is a diagnosis of exclusion, it is not uncommon to have patients state, "No one can figure out what's wrong with me," or, "Other providers have said they didn't know why I have so much pain." Providers, themselves, may be unfamiliar with the disorder and unsure of how to proceed, especially when diagnostic tests have not suggested a reason for the patient's symptoms. Women with signs of vaginismus need to be reassured that their symptoms are real and understand that successful treatment will involve multiple therapies over the course of time.

Follow-Up

Treatment for vaginismus most often involves long-term therapy. This can include a combination of individual and partner counseling, behavioral exercises, neuropathic pain medications, physical therapy, and gradual vaginal dilation and desensitization exercises. If this is a new diagnosis or problem, referrals should be initiated to appropriate health care providers. If the patient has already started treatment, she should be encouraged to continue therapy and attempt pelvic exams at gradual intervals.

FAST FACTS in a NUTSHELL

- Vaginismus occurs in varying degrees, from discomfort to complete closure of the vagina due to spasms.
- Pelvic exams can be completed in stages over the course of many visits.
- Long-term therapy is a mainstay of treatment.

HUMAN TRAFFICKING

Human trafficking can be viewed as a subset of sexual abuse. Commercial sexual exploitation is the most common reason for human trafficking, and adolescents and young women are most at risk. Due to the secretive nature of trafficking, it is difficult to accurately determine the scope of the problem, but it is estimated that more than 14,000 young women and girls are trafficked in the United States each year.

It is very difficult to determine whether a woman is being trafficked. Often there are no definitive signs and the woman will outwardly appear to be just like any other patient. It is important to remember that a woman who is being trafficked is under the control of a pimp who is the gatekeeper to her health care access. Therefore, these women often don't receive routine care. Instead, they present for episodic office visits when there is a problem or concern that is usually related to a gynecologic issue.

The signs of trafficking can be vague and, if they appear individually, may not be enough to raise concern. As with all cases of abuse, the woman's stated history of the illness or injury may not match with the exam findings, or there may be inconsistencies in her account of the problem. A male partner's refusal to leave the woman alone in the exam room or a partner who appears impatient about the length of the office visit may also be indications of control and abuse. Other possible signs of human trafficking include multiple pregnancies and pregnancy terminations, STIs, inconsistent and episodic health care, and overt signs of trauma such as bruising, burns, cuts, and a history of bone fractures. Table 8.2 includes a list of possible signs of human trafficking.

TABLE 8.2 Possible Warning Signs of Human Trafficking

- Homelessness, frequent address changes, inconsistent health care
- Chronic running away (adolescents)
- Presence of an older boyfriend or age disparity in an intimate or sexual relationship
- Tattoos (used to mark victim as property of pimp)
- Signs of violence and/or psychological trauma (including mental illness and suicide attempts)
- STIs, pregnancy, history of abortions
- History of criminal behavior or involvement with youth services
- Substance use/abuse
- Travel with an older male who is not a guardian
- Access to material things that the woman/adolescent cannot afford
- History of family violence
- History of rape or child sexual abuse
- Younger than age 18 and involved in or history of prior prostitution
- Not attending school, frequent absences, or academic failures (adolescents)

Adapted from U.S. Department of Health and Human Services (2009). *Resources: Common health issues seen in victims of human trafficking. Look Beneath the Surface: Restore and Rescue.* Retrieved from http://www.acf.hhs.gov/trafficking/index.html

FAST FACTS in a NUTSHELL

Documentation

- Because there are usually no definitive signs of human trafficking, documentation needs to accurately describe both the patient's history and physical exam findings. Examples:
  - "Recently relocated to area, states unemployed, last gyn exam >2 years ago."
  - "Complaining of pelvic pain, vaginal discharge ×3 weeks."
  - "4 cm yellow bruise on inner aspect of left thigh; pt does not recall injury."

Communication

It is important to establish an open and safe dialogue in all cases of suspected trafficking. There is often a real fear of retaliation from a pimp if the woman's lifestyle is discovered, and women who are trafficked are never sure of who they can trust. Therefore, they are reluctant to disclose a history of abuse. Pimps may threaten with physical harm, deportation if in the country illegally, or harm to family members if the woman divulges the trafficking. Questions for the woman should start with a general health history that includes social aspects, such as work, school, housing, and finances/health insurance. More specific inquiries include questions related to physical and sexual health and safety. Examples of more direct questions are, "Have you been physically or emotionally hurt or threatened by anyone, including a sex partner?" "Have you ever been forced to have sex when you didn't want to?" "Have you ever exchanged sex for drugs, money, or a place to live?"

Follow-Up

Scheduling exam follow-ups can also be challenging. Pimps are typically reluctant to bring these women in for even one visit and can become suspicious if it is recommended that the woman be seen again. If a follow-up exam is scheduled, it is not uncommon for the woman to miss the visit and have contact information that is not valid. These women are moved around frequently and often do not stay in one area long enough to establish consistent health care, although they may come back to the practice after a long absence.

All health care providers should be aware of local recourses in their practice area for patients who are victims or suspected victims of abuse. As with domestic violence, pimps who traffic women use multiple control tactics, including financial control, social isolation, physical control/abuse, and psychological abuse. Leaving a pimp is dangerous and complicated; often these women have no money or personal possessions other than what they are wearing. If the woman is a minor, laws regarding statutory rape and mandatory reporting vary from state to state. All health care providers need to have a list of shelters, abuse hotlines, community advocates, and local law enforcement agencies that can be provided to women.

FAST FACTS in a NUTSHELL

- Sexual trafficking is the most common form of human trafficking.
- Signs of human trafficking are often vague and difficult to determine.
- Gynecologic complaints are common among women who are trafficked.

9

Examining Virginal Women and Premenarchal Children

INTRODUCTION

Women who have never been sexually active and premenarchal children do not require the same screening tests as sexually active adolescents or adult women. Often, gynecologic visits for this group are problem focused, with patients seeking care for specific concerns such as vulvar complaints, vaginitis, abnormal vaginal bleeding, or discomfort. Pelvic exams for these patients should focus on the specific patient concern and be limited to what the patient is able to tolerate.

In this chapter you will learn how to:

1. Apply alternate approaches to performing a pelvic exam on a child.
2. Employ strategies for completing a pelvic exam with virginal women.
3. Recognize situations that warrant specialist referral or delayed/ deferred exam.

VIRGINAL WOMEN

Most young women associate having a pelvic exam with Pap smear screening or obtaining a prescription for contraception. Although annual Pap smear screening is not recommended for women who have never been sexually active, there are other reasons virginal women may require a pelvic exam. The most common reasons for such gynecologic visits include:

- Menstrual cycle abnormalities
- Irregular bleeding
- Vaginal infections
- Pelvic pain

Most often, pelvic exams can be completed on women who have never been sexually active, but some modifications to the exam will increase the patient's comfort and decrease anxiety. Depending on the reason for the exam, it may not be necessary to insert the speculum or perform a bimanual exam. If the patient is complaining of vulvovaginal symptoms such as itching, burning, discharge, or odor, vaginal swabs for wet prep examination and/or cultures/sexually transmitted infection (STI) testing can be collected without using a speculum.

If a speculum exam is necessary, the clinician should consider the following techniques:

- Use a small, narrow speculum to increase the patient's comfort. The hymen often only partially covers the vaginal introitus and will stretch to allow examination.
- A pediatric speculum can be used if the patient is very uncomfortable with the exam.
- With use of either speculum, once inserted, the blades should be opened slowly and only as far as the patient can tolerate.
- If a bimanual exam is warranted, placing only one finger in the vagina instead of two will decrease discomfort for the patient.

FAST FACTS in a NUTSHELL

Documentation

- The clinician should document the woman's ability to tolerate the exam. Examples:
  - "Long, narrow speculum used and able to visualize cervix."
  - Patient tolerated exam fairly well.
  - "Limited bimanual exam performed with one finger."

Communication

Women who have never been sexually active often have anxiety and misconceptions about the pelvic exam. The extent of the exam will depend on their history and symptoms. Women should be reassured that they will still be a virgin after the exam. Women who use tampons are often less uncomfortable with the exam and it may be helpful to ask the patient if she has ever been able to insert a tampon prior to beginning. Let women know that they can request to have the exam stopped at any time due to anxiety or discomfort.

Follow-Up

In the context of a normal exam, no specific follow-up may be required. If pathology is suspected and the exam is very limited by the woman's discomfort, an ultrasound, endometrial biopsy, hysterosalpingogram, or other diagnostic testing can be ordered as necessary and as indicated.

FAST FACTS in a NUTSHELL

- Choose a narrow, Pederson type speculum.
- Consider a bimanual exam with one finger.

CHILDREN AND PREMENARCHAL PATIENTS

In order to successfully perform a gynecologic exam of a young child or a child who has not yet reached menarche, the clinician must approach the exam differently than with an adult. Some special considerations to keep in mind when working with very young children and premenarchal girls include:

- The exam cannot be hurried or rushed, and the clinician must be gentle, patient, and understanding of both the child's and parent's anxiety.
- Schedule extra time for the exam, especially if the child is new to the practice and not familiar with the staff and office.
- Place all instruments out of sight.
- The clinician should consider removing the lab coat.

Obtaining a history from a child can be challenging, especially with very young children. Parents will often provide the majority of the child's health history and reason for the visit. Even verbal and social children will often be extremely quiet in a new setting when they are nervous and anxious. For some children, pictures or dolls can be helpful tools to determine level of pain or location of a problem. Crying, fussing, and clinging to a parent are all normal childhood responses to fear and discomfort and should be anticipated during the visit.

Tanner Staging

Knowledge of child growth and development is necessary for any health care providers who work with children. Pubertal changes and maturation occur in a sequential, predictable manner and are visible through the appearance of secondary sex characteristics. The average age for first appearance

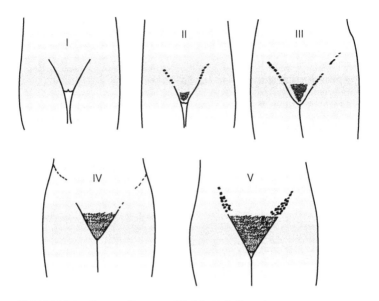

FIGURE 9.1   Tanner Stages of Pubic Hair Development.

of pubic hair varies depending on race and ethnicity, but typically ranges from 9 to 10 years of age.

The staging system for pubertal development that is most commonly used is referred to as Tanner stages (Figure 9.1). For females, these stages describe breast and pubic hair development, but for the purposes of this chapter the focus will be on pubic hair changes only. The stages range from 1 to 5, with 1 representing a preadolescent with no pubic hair and 5 representing the pubic hair pattern of an adult woman.

Tanner Stages of Pubic Hair in Girls

Stage 1: Prepubertal (velus hair similar to abdominal wall)

Stage 2: Sparse growth of long, slightly pigmented hair, straight or curled, along labia

Stage 3: Darker, coarser, and more curly hair, spreading sparsely over pubic area

Stage 4: Adult-type hair, covering smaller area with no spread to medial surface of thighs

Stage 5: Adult in type and quantity, with horizontal distribution (adapted from childgrowthfoundation.org/psm_tanner_stages.htm)

Examining Children

It is very important to emphasize that the majority of the exam will be "just looking," without having to touch. Use of stirrups will be determined based on age, understanding, and anxiety level of the child. Older children will most likely be able to tolerate positioning with stirrups. For young children, alternate positions are best. The child can remain on the parent's lap in a frog-legged position, or this position can also be used on an exam table if the child doesn't fit comfortably in the parent's lap. A lateral side-lying position is also an option if this makes the child more comfortable. Undressing completely and changing into an exam gown will often increase anxiety and therefore the child should only remove clothing that is necessary to complete the exam.

Gynecologic exams on children are primarily external. Significant gynecologic problems in this age group are rare and the vast majority of complaints are related to vulvovaginitis. Often the vagina can be visualized by asking the child to cough or bear down. Any specimens can be collected from the vaginal introitus with a small swab without using a speculum. Older children who are closer to menarche may be able to tolerate a speculum exam. In this situation, the smallest speculum should be used. A nasal otoscope may also be used when the smallest speculum is still too large.

FAST FACTS in a NUTSHELL

Documentation

- Documentation should include reference to positioning during the exam. Examples:
  - "Patient examined frog-legged on exam table, supported by mother."
- Information should be provided about exam findings. Examples:
  - "External vulvar erythema of the labia minora and majora, present bilaterally."
  - "No evidence of foreign body at introitus with coughing."

Communication

When performing an exam on a child, communication will alternate between the child and parent. If the child is a toddler with limited language, the majority of the history and symptoms will be elicited from the parent. Although you can obtain a large portion of the history from the parents, children can help give concrete facts about symptoms and their location, especially if they are school-aged. Make your questions short and direct and include language that the child will understand. Parents can provide you with terms they use for different body parts and bodily functions. When talking, you should be sitting at eye level with the child and allow adequate time for the child to give her answer.

Follow-Up

If necessary, plans for follow-up care should be made after a discussion of exam findings with the child's parents. If a speculum exam is necessary because pathology or a foreign body is suspected, the clinician should consider a referral to a pediatric gynecologist, especially for very young children. Exams of this nature may need to be conducted under anesthesia or ultrasound guidance. In cases of suspected child sexual abuse, referrals should be initiated for a sexual assault forensic exam and notification of local child services and law enforcement agencies.

FAST FACTS in a NUTSHELL

- Gynecologic exams on children consist primarily of inspection of the external genitalia and most do not require a speculum.
- If a more detailed internal exam is necessary, referral to a pediatric gynecologist should be considered.
- If the history reveals possible sexual abuse of a child, immediate referral to a pediatric sexual assault nurse examiner is recommended.

For further information related to specific pelvic exam challenges and potential resolutions, please see Appendix A.

10

Techniques Useful When Examining Overweight, Multiparous, or Physically Challenged Women

INTRODUCTION

Examining women who are obese, multiparous, or have physical conditions that limit their mobility can be very challenging for both the clinician and the patient. Often, adjustments need to be made to the physical office space and equipment. Extra time and preparation for the exam will increase the patient's comfort and chances for a successful exam. Additionally, extra staff may be needed to assist with transfers, positioning, safety, and specimen collection.

In this chapter you will learn how to:

1. Identify specific challenges to performing a pelvic exam on patients who are obese.
2. Identify physical changes that are common with multiparity.
3. List strategies to accommodate women who are physically challenged.

OBESITY

Obese women are less likely to receive routine gynecologic care than are women with a body mass index (BMI) in the healthy range. Weight bias and fear of judgment may contribute to avoidance of gynecologic care. Exam tables, equipment, and gowns are often inadequate, especially for morbidly obese women. The clinician needs to be sensitive to the needs of overweight women and adjust her/his exam techniques accordingly.

Impaired mobility may be the first challenge when working with obese patients. Often, positioning on the exam table can be difficult. Exam tables are narrow and women who are significantly overweight may feel as if they will fall off. Once on the table, obese women may have less ability to flex and rotate their hips when positioning in the stirrups.

Clinicians may need staff assistance when performing the pelvic exam. Employing a few helpful techniques serves to reduce or avoid patient embarrassment. These include the following:

- The patient's thighs may need to be retracted when in the stirrups. An assistant can help gently hold back any skin folds that are obscuring the vulva and vagina.
- Obese women often have excess vaginal skin and tissue that can make visualizing the cervix challenging. Using a larger speculum and palpating the cervix prior to inserting the speculum will help facilitate the exam.
- Asking the patient to flex her hips upward may also bring the cervix into a better position for viewing.
- Once the speculum is inserted and opened, it may still be difficult to visualize the cervix. Speculums lack lateral support, and thus the vaginal sidewalls can collapse inward and obscure the view of the cervix. In this situation, cutting off the closed end of a condom or glove finger and slipping this over the closed speculum blades is very helpful. When opened, the sheath assists in holding back any redundant tissue that may block the cervix.

Bimanual exams are often less sensitive due to excess adipose tissue, especially if the woman has a large abdominal pannus. If you are having difficulty palpating through extra lower abdominal tissue, the patient may be able to help by holding back the skin in this area. If you are unable to adequately assess the uterus and ovaries and the patient and/or you as the clinician suspect pathology, ultrasound evaluation of the pelvic organs may be useful option.

════ *FAST FACTS in a NUTSHELL*

Documentation
- Any difficulty with the exam or inability to adequately assess internal organs should be documented. Examples:
  - "Exam limited by abdominal obesity."
  - "Unable to assess uterus and ovaries due to body habitus and/or abdominal obesity."

Communication

Obese and overweight women often face societal discrimination due to their body size. Many avoid routine health care due to anxiety over being weighed and fear of judgment by health care providers. Statements such as, "You need to lose weight," or, "Your BMI is too high" are unhelpful and often frustrating to women. Care should be taken to discuss weight-related issues in terms of concern over actual or potential health consequences.

Statements that show understanding and concern regarding patient complaints are far more effective than general declarations about obesity. For example, stating, "Heavy menstrual periods can be one complication of obesity. Reducing your weight will often help reduce bleeding. Let's talk about a plan to set weight loss goals and monitor your menstrual cycles," shows that you understand the significance of the problem and you care about finding a solution. It is far more effective than saying, "You need to lose weight to help decrease the bleeding."

If the exam is limited by obesity, the patient should be told in a clear, nonjudgmental manner. Patients have a right and responsibility to understand the findings of the health care visit. "Due to the shape and size of your body, I wasn't able to feel your uterus and ovaries" is a direct and factual statement about the limitations of the exam. This will allow for discussion about whether further evaluation is necessary.

Follow-Up

A decision to recommend additional evaluation of the obese patient will depend on presenting symptoms and exam findings. In the presence of normal menstrual cycles and no gynecologic-related complaints, a limited exam may not require any follow-up other than reevaluation at the next scheduled health care visit. If the patient presents with complaints of menstrual irregularities, pain, or other symptoms that suggest a gynecologic origin, then additional evaluation is warranted. Most often this can be accomplished with pelvic ultrasound.

FAST FACTS in a NUTSHELL

- Using a wider, larger speculum may help bring the cervix into view.
- Palpating the cervix prior to inserting the speculum will assist with location.
- Asking the patient to flex/lift her hips up can change the position of the cervix.
- Placing a condom or finger of a glove with one end cut off over the speculum can hold back the lateral walls of the vagina and allow the cervix to be seen.
- Placing a towel or small pillow under the patient's hips may also help the clinician visualize the patient's cervix.

MULTIPARITY

The main challenges associated with multiparity are related to lax muscles in the vaginal wall or pelvic floor. Childbirth and multiple deliveries can weaken pelvic muscles and contribute to uterine prolapse, cystocele, and rectocele formation. When these conditions occur it is often difficult to locate the cervix because landmarks can change and bulging in the vaginal walls may block visualization of the cervix. Additionally, after pregnancy and delivery, the cervix may move to a posterior position, which can make it more difficult to see with an average-sized speculum.

Locating/palpating the cervix manually prior to speculum insertion will help identify position and assist in determining whether the cervix is located posteriorly. Some helpful techniques include the following:

- If the cervix appears to be posterior, use a longer speculum for adequate visualization and specimen collection.
- If weakened vaginal muscles or bulging from the bladder or rectum obscures the cervix, proceed as you would with obese women and include a combination of repositioning the patient with her hips tilted upward and placing a sheath over the speculum blades to hold back any tissue that is blocking the cervix.

FAST FACTS in a NUTSHELL

Documentation
- It is important to document the location of pelvic anatomy. Examples:
  - "Parous os, posterior. Cervix visualized with long speculum."
  - "Mild uterine prolapse, cervix located at mid-vagina."
  - "Moderate uterine prolapse, cervix at vaginal introitus."

Communication

Multiparous patients should have the findings of their exam communicated in a straightforward manner, using correct anatomical terms for anatomy and physical findings. Care should be taken to avoid suggesting that childbirth has "stretched out" the vagina or caused their uterus, bladder, or rectum to "fall." Patients should be reassured that pregnancy and delivery may change the shape and location of the cervix, but that this is a normal and expected finding that does not need any intervention. The presence of a cystocele, rectocele, or uterine prolapse should be discussed in terms of possible symptoms, side effects, and whether the degree of muscle prolapse requires further evaluation and intervention.

Follow-Up

Further evaluation is determined by the severity of any abnormal findings and whether the patient is experiencing discomfort or side effects. There are many options to strengthen pelvic floor muscle tone. Women can be taught to perform Kegel exercises by contracting (squeezing) the muscles normally used to stop urine flow. Muscles should be contracted for a few seconds and then released. This is repeated 10 to 15 times. This cycle of contracting and releasing the pelvic floor muscles should be done at least 3 times throughout the day. Additionally, patients can be referred to physical therapy to specifically target the pelvic floor. Surgical evaluation should be considered if the uterus is prolapsed to the vaginal introitus or beyond, or if urinary and fecal incontinence is significantly decreasing the quality of life and interfering with daily activities.

============*FAST FACTS in a NUTSHELL*

- Palpating the cervix prior to inserting the speculum will assist with location.
- Placing a condom or finger of a glove with one end cut off over the speculum can hold back the lateral walls of the vagina and allow the examiner to visualize the cervix.
- Using a wider, longer speculum may help bring the cervix into view.

PHYSICALLY CHALLENGED

Women who are disabled or physically challenged face multiple challenges when accessing health care. This population has the same gynecologic health care needs as all women; they need access to timely gynecologic and breast exams in addition to their special health care needs. However, their chronic health care needs related to their disability often take precedence and routine gynecologic care and pelvic exams may be neglected.

Many of the challenges in providing gynecologic care to a woman with a disability are related to the physical space of the health care practice. Exam rooms are often small and maneuvering with a wheelchair, scooter, or other assistive devices such as a walker can be extremely difficult. The exam room may need to be rearranged or furniture such as extra chairs may need to be temporarily removed to accommodate larger equipment such as a wheelchair.

An exam table with a hydraulic lift is ideal for patients who have mobility impairment. Most practices are only equipped with standard, nonadjustable exam tables that are too high for patients to safely transfer from a wheelchair. If this exam table is not available, health care personnel must be aware of how to assist patients with physical disabilities onto standard exam tables. Once on the examination table, a woman with mobility impairment may need handrails and adjustable foot rests in order to stay safely on the table. Padded or strapped stirrups can increase comfort, especially for women with leg spasticity, weakness, contractures, and/or tremors. Women with impaired mobility should be booked for longer appointments and at a time when extra staff are available to provide assistance and ensure safety.

Prior to the exam, the woman should empty her bladder either on her own or by intermittent bladder catheterization. Many women with physical disabilities cannot comfortably assume the lithotomy position that is traditionally used for pelvic exams. This position will be difficult for many women with paralysis, muscle weakness, spasticity, low muscle tone, and conditions that cause chronic pain and inflammation. Alternative positions should be considered based upon the individual woman and her specific disability. Sidelying, knee-chest, diamond shape (knees abducted and feet together, no stirrups), legs straight and extended into a V shape, and M shape (feet flat on exam table, no stirrups) are all possibilities from which women and providers can choose. See Figure 10.1, Illustrations of alternate positioning.

Communication

Although many women with physical disabilities come to health care visits with a partner, family member, or other caregiver, it should not be assumed that the disabled woman is unable to speak for herself. Communication with women who are physically challenged should always be specifically directed to them. Other support persons may be present

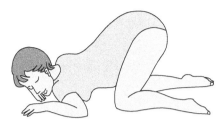

Knee-chest position

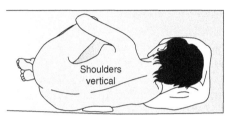

Shoulders
vertical

Lateral recumbent position

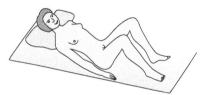

Dorsal recumbent position

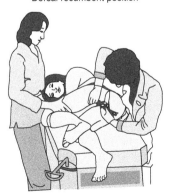

The physically accessible position

FIGURE 10.1 Illustrations of alternate positioning.

FAST FACTS in a NUTSHELL

Documentation

- Always document precautions used to ensure safety. Examples:
  - "Two-person assist for transfer from wheelchair (or chair) to exam table; table set and locked to lowest position."
  - "Medical assistant present during exam and to assist with positioning on and off exam table."
- Documentation should include exam findings and the patient's ability to tolerate the exam. Examples:
  - "Patient unable to place legs in stirrups. Exam performed with legs flat on exam table extended into a V shape."
  - "Pelvic exam limited by pain and muscle spasticity."
  - "Patient tolerated exam well without hypotension or syncope."

during conversations but should not be used as interpreters or health care decision-makers unless this is explicitly stated by the patient.

Communication should flow normally as it would with patients who are not disabled. Let the patient know the office staff and you are available for assistance but also don't assume they are unable to care for themselves. If necessary, ask direct, matter-of-fact questions if there is something of which you are unsure. If assistive equipment needs to be moved in the exam room due to space constraints, you should seek permission prior to relocating any devices. Moving equipment without the patient's consent may place it out of reach and result in a risk for fall or injury.

It should never be assumed that a woman who is physically challenged is not sexually active solely due to her disability. These women need *to be asked* the same sexual history screening questions as women who are not disabled (see Chapter 1 for how to conduct a sexual history). If sexually active, type of sexual activity, number of partners, risk for pregnancy and STIs, and any reproductive health concerns need to be assessed. Asking direct questions such as, "Do you have any questions or concerns about your sexual health that I can help you with today?" will allow for open dialogue that will lay the foundation for a thorough gynecologic exam.

Follow-Up

During the course of the visit it may become apparent that follow-up is recommended based on exam findings. Your assessment may reveal complications related to the disability such as pain, muscle atrophy, skin breakdown, or excoriation from prosthetic devices. If any of your findings are chronic problems, the patient should be advised to continue regular health care and monitor for worsening symptoms. New-onset symptoms, whether related to the disability or gynecologic origin, should be assessed more immediately. A plan for follow-up should be agreed on with the patient and referrals implemented as necessary. Routine screening, such as mammograms and blood work, should be scheduled with facilities that are able to easily accommodate women with physical challenges.

FAST FACTS in a NUTSHELL

- Preparation of the patient, staff, space, and equipment are all necessary to ensure a safe and adequate exam for women with physical disabilities.
- Be familiar with alternate positions for performing a pelvic exam.

For further information related to specific pelvic exam challenges and potential resolutions, please see Appendix A.

II

Special Considerations When Examining the Menopausal and Elder Woman

INTRODUCTION

Performing a gynecologic exam on menopausal and elderly women requires special skills and knowledge of the physical, psychological, and social changes pertinent to this population. These include awareness of atrophic and age-related genital and pelvic exam findings. In addition, practitioners must be sensitive to additional changes associated with aging, including decreased mobility, existing chronic health conditions, cognitive impairment, and impairment in eyesight and hearing.

In this chapter you will learn how to:

1. Identify normal aging changes of the vulva and vagina.
2. Identify atrophic changes associated with menopause.
3. Recognize challenges to examining postmenopausal women and identify approaches to managing the pelvic exam.

EXAMINING THE MENOPAUSAL AND ELDER WOMAN

Estrogen deficiency is present in all menopausal women. The genital skin and vaginal lining are estrogen dependent. Therefore, menopause and aging produce changes in the urogenital system that includes a shift in vaginal flora/environment, a thinning of the vaginal tissue, and loss of elasticity. These changes increase the likelihood that the pelvic exam will be uncomfortable. As a result, clinicians must approach the pelvic exam with care and sensitivity.

Medical problems associated with menopause may include (Carcio & Secor, 2010, p. 352):

- Cardiovascular conditions such as heart attack or stroke
- Diabetes mellitus: metabolic syndrome
- Osteoporosis or osteopenia
- Asthma
- Cancers of the reproductive tract
- Sexually transmitted infections (STIs)
- Pregnancy/infertility
- Distressing vasomotor symptoms (VMS)
- Adverse effects of traditional and alternative therapies
- Gallbladder disease

AGE-RELATED AND ATROPHIC CHANGES

Certain changes associated with the loss of estrogen are identifiable when performing a gynecologic exam on an elderly or older woman. Age-related changes of the external genitalia include thinning and graying of pubic hair, and thinning and dryness of external genital skin.

Internally, atrophic vaginitis may be evident. Inflammation from loss of estrogen can manifest as vaginal dryness, tissue pallor or erythema, loss of overall vaginal tone, decreased

TABLE 11.1 Comparative Assessment Findings: Atrophic Vaginitis Versus Bacterial Vaginosis (BV, or *Gardnerella*)

Atrophic Vaginitis	Bacterial Vaginosis
Inspection Tissue is friable erythema Lesions, condyloma Scant, colorless discharge Sparse, brittle pubic hair Shrinking of the labia minora Possible inflammation of the vulva Vulva may be erythematous and edematous Excoriation (from vulvar pruritus)	*Inspection* Little or no inflammation of vaginal epithelium Assoc with a pink, healthy cervix [Note: "Strawberry cervix" is seen with cervicitis due to *T. vaginalis*; red, edematous, friable cervix is associated with *Chlamydia* trachomatis]
Speculum Exam Thin, pale, erythematous, friable vaginal epithelium Decreased or absent vaginal rugae Scant, thin, variable, non-malodorous discharge Vaginal pH greater than 4.6 Amine test negative Microscopy: Negative for clue cells, positive for WBCs, and immature epithelial cells. Also referred to as an abnormal maturation index diagnostic of atrophic vaginitis.	*Speculum exam* Homogeneous, white, adherent vaginal discharge Vaginal pH greater than 4.6 (normal is 5.5–7.0) (take smear for testing from the lateral walls of the vagina, not from the cervix) Fishy, amine-like odor from vaginal fluid before and/or after missing it with 10% potassium hydroxide (positive whiff test) [Note: Semen releases the vaginal amines; therefore, there is an increased odor after intercourse] Presence of "clue cells" (squamous vaginal epithelial cells covered with bacteria, causing a stippled or granular appearance, and ragged, "moth-eaten" borders)

Adapted with permission from Cash, J. C., & Glass, C.A. (2010). *Family practice guidelines* (2nd ed., p. 321). New York, NY: Springer Publishing Company.

vaginal rugae, and loss of tissue elasticity. Cystocele and recto-cele may be present. Discharge associated with atrophic vagi-nitis may be scant or copious, thin or thick, white or yellow, and may be associated with odor. The cervix of postmeno-pausal women may also lose some definition and appear flat and short. Friability and bleeding with Pap smears are com-mon, and often the cervical os is stenotic, which can make endocervical sampling for Pap testing challenging.

Age-related changes are also evident during the bimanual pelvic exam. Overall, pelvic reproductive organs atrophy. The uterus may be small and less mobile. If the uterus is enlarged, this may suggest pregnancy (if premenopausal) or pathol-ogy such as uterine hyperplasia, fibroids, or carcinoma. The ovaries of a postmenopausal or elderly woman are gener-ally not palpable, but, if palpable, the clinician should rule out pathology by ultrasound, CA125 and possible consultation/ referral to a gynecologist. A comparative summary of findings associated with atrophic vaginitis and other vaginal infec-tions can be found in Table 11.1.

THE PELVIC EXAM OF THE POSTMENOPAUSAL WOMAN

The atrophic changes produced by the loss of estrogen can make the pelvic exam uncomfortable for the patient and challenging for the clinician. Age-related changes such as decreased range of motion, arthritis, and mobility impairments can limit patient po-sitioning on the exam table. Any cognitive impairments and/or sensory impairments of sight and hearing can decrease the ability to follow directions and cooperate with the exam process. Assis-tance from additional staff may be needed to help with position-ing on the exam table, patient safety, leg support, and obtaining specimens. If mobility and flexibility are extremely limited, the provider can perform a partial exam with the patient in the left lateral position with the right knee flexed (Sim's position).

Gentleness cannot be overemphasized, especially during the speculum exam. Quick insertion of the speculum and vigorous movements can be painful and damaging to thin, friable tissues. The blades of the speculum should be opened slowly and carefully to avoid vaginal tissue damage, irritation, and bleeding. Using a smaller Pederson speculum with narrower blades is often more comfortable for older women. If vaginal dryness is making speculum insertion very painful or impossible, placing a small amount of lubricant on the tip of the blades will make insertion and movement of the speculum easier. If atrophy is so significant that the pelvic exam is impossible, local application of topical estrogen (either externally or vaginal) can be tried for 2 to 4 weeks (or longer, if necessary) and the exam attempted again after treatment.

After menopause, the cervix may lose its landmarks and become difficult to visualize, as it shortens and becomes flush with the vaginal walls. In addition, the cervical os may become smaller and stenosed, making it difficult to obtain an adequate sample for Pap smear testing. If Pap smear testing is warranted, you should insert the cytobrush approximately 1 cm into the os or as far as possible without force or trauma to the cervical canal. If a traditional Pap smear cannot be obtained, a blind Pap with HPV DNA testing can be considered, especially for women who are at low risk for cervical cancer. Lack of estrogen makes the cervix friable and associated bleeding with cervical and endocervical sampling is not uncommon.

Other aspects of the pelvic exam may also be challenging. Bimanual exam may be limited by not only atrophic changes but also central obesity, which is common in menopausal women. Due to atrophy and decreased elasticity, the bimanual exam may be uncomfortable. You may only be able to introduce one finger into the vagina. Palpate the uterus for shape and size. The uterus usually decreases in size after menopause due to atrophy. Therefore, enlargement or irregular shape requires additional evaluation. A summary of exam findings for women using and not using local estrogen can be found in Table 11.2.

TABLE 11.2 Assessment Findings of the Menopausal Woman: Using and Not Using Local Estrogen

Findings of Area Assessed

Findings if NOT Using Local Estrogen	Findings if Using Local Estrogen
External Genitalia	
Thinning and/or graying of pubic hair	Tissues pink, moist
Tissue pallor	Landmarks stable
Loss of architectural features (landmarks)	Elastic, durable tissues
Erythema	Nontender
Easily traumatized (lesions or fissures)	No caruncle
Tenderness	Introitus normal size, with moderate tone
Urethral caruncle (small friable polyp)	Stable or improving cystocele, rectocele
Introital shrinkage or laxity	
Cystocele	
Rectocele	
Vagina	
Introital laxity	Improving introital tone
Loss of rugae (flattening)	Rugations present
Loss of tone with Kegel and Valsalva maneuver	Improved tone with Kegel and Valsalva maneuver
Shortening of vagina	Normal vaginal size and elasticity
Cervix	
Erythema	Pink
Lesions	No lesions
Friability	Nonfriable
Bleeding	Nontender
Tenderness	Less flattening with extended use
Flattening	Normal cervical os size (with continued use)
Shortening	
Stenosis of cervical os (small)	
Uterus	
Size and shape may be asymmetrical (associated with fibroids that shrink in menopause)	Local estrogen does not influence uterus size or shape
Diffuse enlargement (associated with pathology such as hyperplasia)	Systemic estrogen for hot flashes may cause fibroids to grow
Tenderness	
Sometimes fibroids	

(continued)

TABLE 11.2 *(continued)*	
Findings if NOT Using Local Estrogen	**Findings if Using Local Estrogen**
Pelvic Floor	
Cystocele	Stable or improving cystocele,
Rectocele	rectocele
Diminished introital tone with Kegel and Valsalva maneuver	Improved introital tone with Kegel and Valsalva maneuver
Ovaries	
Not palpable	Not palpable

Adapted with permission from Carcio, H. A., & Secor, M. C. (2010). *Advanced health assessment of women: Clinical skills and procedures* (2nd ed., p. 355). New York, NY: Springer Publishing Company.

HEALTH ISSUES OF OLDER WOMEN

In addition to the specific gynecologic changes associated with menopause and aging, older women can experience a wide variety of health issues related to the aging process. These chronic illnesses can have a significant impact on quality of life and are a major contributor to the morbidity and mortality of older women.

- Cardiovascular disease is a broad heading that includes specific illnesses such as hypertension, cerebral vascular accidents (CVAs), congestive heart failure (CHF), and coronary artery disease (CAD). Cardiovascular disease remains the leading cause of death among women. Symptoms of acute myocardial infarction (MI) in women often present as more subtle symptoms of left arm and jaw discomfort rather than the substernal chest pain experienced by men.
- Cancer is still primarily a disease associated with aging; the vast majority of all cancers are diagnosed at age 55 or older. Breast, lung, and colorectal cancers are

the most common cancers among women, with lung cancer having the highest mortality rate. Strategies for prevention and early diagnosis focus on healthy lifestyle changes and routine screening, such as mammograms and colonoscopy.

- Diabetes in older women is primarily adult onset or type 2 diabetes mellitus. This form of diabetes is characterized by a decreased sensitivity to insulin. Type 2 diabetes is often preventable with weight reduction and increased physical activity, and is treated with lifestyle and dietary changes and medication. As the presence of diabetes increases the risk for cardiovascular disease, women should be strongly encouraged to closely manage their diabetes.

- Osteoporosis, the loss of bone density, is estimated to affect up to 20% of women over the age of 50 and is a major contributor to hip fractures in older women. The decline in estrogen that occurs with menopause is the leading cause of osteoporosis in women. Fractures, especially of the hip and vertebra, are often the first symptom of the disease and cause significant morbidity and mortality among older women.

LABORATORY EVALUATION OF MENOPAUSAL AND ELDER WOMEN

There is no specific set of "menopause labs" that is appropriate for every woman. The decision to assess certain laboratory functions will be made based on each individual woman's history and presenting symptoms. Some laboratory tests to consider are specific to the menopause transition, while others relate to diseases that are more common with aging and loss of estrogen and progesterone.

- Serum follicle-stimulating hormone (FSH) is the test most commonly associated with diagnosing menopause, but not without controversy. A normal FSH range for menstruating women is typically between 4 and 21 mIU/mL, although this may differ slightly among laboratories. When FSH levels rise above 30, women are considered to be in menopause. A clinical history of 12 consecutive months of amenorrhea is diagnostic of menopause and FSH levels are not needed to confirm clinical data.
- Thyroid-stimulating hormone (TSH) is commonly measured to evaluate thyroid functioning. The incidence of hypothyroidism increases with age and it is estimated that up to 10% of women experience hypothyroidism by age 65. TSH is often measured to rule out a thyroid disorder as the cause of irregular menses and amenorrhea that occur with menopause.
- Estradiol is primarily made by the ovaries and decreases as ovarian function declines and eventually stops with menopause. There is a wide range for estradiol levels depending on menstrual cycle phase, but levels less than 30 pg/mL are associated with menopause.
- Luteinizing hormone (LH) is released by the pituitary gland and in menstruating women increases during the middle of the menstrual cycle to trigger ovulation. Normal levels range from 5 to 25 IU/L. During menopause, LH levels rise as ovarian function declines and the ovaries are less responsive to LH surges.
- Other laboratory tests to consider as women age are fasting lipid profile (FLP) and blood glucose. These tests are important in assessing risk factors for cardiovascular disease. Bone mineral density (BMD) testing and mammogram screenings should be performed according to established guidelines and individual risk factors.

===== *FAST FACTS in a NUTSHELL*

Documentation
- Documentation should focus on physical findings related to menopause. Examples:
  - "Vagina atrophic, pale dry; decreased rugation."
  - "Uterus small, smooth, mobile, nontender; ovaries nonpalpable."

Communication

Women should be reassured that the transition to menopause is a normal and expected life transition and not a pathologic state. Not all women will experience physical and emotional symptoms related to menopause. Anticipatory guidance will help dispel myths and misconceptions about menopause and aging. If women are concerned about menopause symptoms, they should be informed about pharmacologic and alternative therapies that are available to decrease discomfort, primarily from vasomotor instability.

Follow-Up

There is no specific follow-up required if the exam is normal and the patient has no immediate concerns. Menstrual calendars can be a useful tool to help women track their menstrual cycles as changes occur during the transition to menopause. A pelvic ultrasound can be considered to assess pelvic anatomy if the exam is suggestive of uterine fibroids or an ovarian mass. If menstrual bleeding is excessive, there is a concern about hyperplasia, or the patient complains of abnormal vaginal bleeding especially after menopause (occurring after 12 months since LMP), the patient should have an endometrial biopsy or be referred for one. A transvaginal ultrasound may also be considered.

FAST FACTS in a NUTSHELL

- Having the patient apply daily estrogen to the external genital area for 4 to 6 weeks prior to the exam may decrease discomfort by thickening and increasing elasticity of the vaginal tissues.
- Using a long, narrow Pederson or pediatric speculum will decrease discomfort.
- For patients who are extremely uncomfortable, applying a small amount of lidocaine gel to the vaginal introitus a few minutes prior to the exam may be beneficial.
- Use slow, gentle movements to decrease the chance of trauma with the exam.

For further information related to specific pelvic exam challenges and potential resolutions, please see Appendix A.

12

Care of the Woman Who Has Experienced Female Genital Mutilation

INTRODUCTION

Female genital mutilation (FGM), also called female circumcision or female cutting, is defined by the World Health Organization (WHO) as any procedure that involves partial or complete removal the external female genitalia or injury to the female genitals for nonmedical reasons. It is estimated that 100 to 140 million women worldwide have experienced some type of FGM and millions more are at risk. Although this practice occurs globally, it is most common in African, Middle Eastern, and some Asian countries. FGM is illegal in the United States, but practitioners may encounter women who have immigrated to the United States after having the procedure in their native country as a child.

In this chapter you will learn how to:

1. Identify different classifications of FGM.
2. Recognize the long-term sequelae of FGM.
3. Employ strategies for performing a pelvic exam after FGM.

131

CLASSIFICATION OF FGM

The WHO has classified FGM into four categories that are based on the extent of damage to the genitalia.

- Type I involves removal of the clitoris and/or prepuce.
- Type II involves removal of the clitoris plus partial or total removal of the labia minora and possibly the labia majora.
- Type III mutilation narrows the vaginal opening by sealing over the orifice with tissue from the labia minora or majora and may also include removal of the clitoris. This level of mutilation always involves suturing that reduces the size of the vaginal introitus and often the urethral opening, as well.
- Type IV includes any other harmful procedures to the female genitals that are not medically necessary. Examples include piercing, burning, scarring, or other nontherapeutic and unnecessary incisions.

FAST FACTS in a NUTSHELL

The level of anatomical alteration will differ depending on the type of FGM.

LONG-TERM SEQUELAE OF FGM

The majority of FGM occurs in young girls prior to or at the onset of puberty. Therefore, most practitioners in the United States will not experience acute cases. Rather, they will encounter women in the clinical setting long after the procedure has been performed and healing has occurred. These encounters may occur as part of a routine visit, or women may seek care due to an ongoing complication from the procedure.

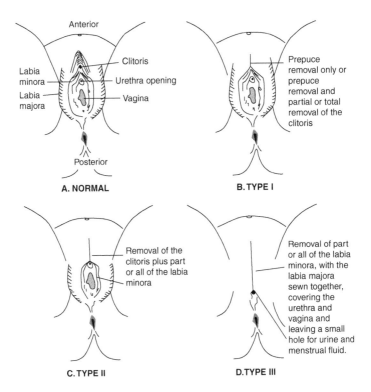

FIGURE 12.1 Female Genital Mutilation classifications.

- With type I and II FGM procedures, the level of scarring will vary depending on the individual woman and the conditions and instruments used in the initial procedure (Figure 12.1).
  - Possible physical symptoms include large keloid scars and epidermal inclusion cysts. Abscess formation along the scar line will present as a painful enlarging mass in the genital area.
  - Some possible presenting symptoms include complaints of friable or pruritic vulvar skin that is prone to excoriation and infection and dyspareunia.

- With type III FGM, a common gynecologic complaint is dysmenorrhea and symptoms related to the narrowed vaginal opening. These can be grouped into the following categories:
  - Narrowing of the vaginal opening.
    - Hematocolpos. This buildup of menstrual blood in the vagina results from mechanical obstruction of menstruation. Women with this condition may present with complaints of intermittent abdominal pain, constipation, urinary retention, and complaints of vulvar pressure and bulging in the vaginal area.
    - Sexual problems. Women may relate unsuccessful attempts at vaginal intercourse, infertility, sexual dysfunction, and severe dyspareunia.
    - History of chronic vaginitis and pruritus.
  - Narrowing of the urethral opening. Women with this condition might relate a variety of urinary complaints, including prolonged voiding time, history of urinary tract infections, weak urinary flow, and dysuria.

PERFORMING A PELVIC EXAM AFTER FGM

Performing a pelvic exam on a woman who has undergone FGM requires extra time and sensitivity. A thorough reproductive history should include a discussion of any previous or current sexual activity or attempts at sexual activity. Depending on the level of alteration and scarring, successful vaginal penetration may not be possible or may be possible only in the presence of severe dyspareunia. Characteristics of menstrual and urinary flow will help determine if vaginal and urinary openings have been significantly narrowed. The clinician should also inquire about any history of vaginal pain, itching, or sexually transmitted infections (STIs).

An external exam will reveal altered anatomy and scarring, and clinical anatomical landmarks may be difficult to identify or completely absent. Determining how much the woman understands about the level of genital modification will help the clinician guide the flow of the pelvic exam. The type of FGM will guide how to proceed with an internal exam.

FAST FACTS in a NUTSHELL

Depending on the age of the woman when FGM was performed, she may or may not have a complete understanding of the extent of her injuries. If she was raised in an environment where all women have experienced FGM, she may have never seen unaltered female anatomy.

If the vaginal introitus is extremely narrow, pelvic exams may be difficult or impossible. A thin adult speculum or a pediatric speculum may be necessary when obtaining a Pap smear. If the woman cannot tolerate even the smallest speculum, the Pap smear and other cervical and vaginal samples (for STIs and vaginitis) can be collected with a blind sweep. STIs and pregnancy may also be ruled out by urine testing. Assessing internal pelvic organs with a bimanual exam may also be very limited or impossible due to pain; in this situation, a pelvic ultrasound may be helpful.

Strategies to help reduce discomfort during the exam include:

- Encouraging the patient to employ the deep breathing technique
- Use of slow, gentle movements by the examiner
- Application of topical lubricants and lidocaine to the area prior to the exam

While such strategies can be effective in reducing discomfort during a pelvic exam, these approaches may be of limited effectiveness in the presence of significantly altered anatomy.

==*FAST FACTS in a NUTSHELL*

Documentation

- In addition to documenting any adverse symptoms, it is important to describe exam findings in great detail. Although it may not be possible to determine the exact level of FGM, a clear description of anatomical findings is necessary to establish a plan of care. Examples:
  - "Clitoris absent, well-healed scar."
  - "Labia minora absent, urethral and vaginal openings patent without narrowing or scar tissue."
- The patient's response to the pelvic exam should be noted. Examples:
  - "Able to insert narrow speculum but unable to open blades due to patient discomfort."
  - "Bimanual exam limited by vaginal stricture and patient discomfort."

Communication

Culturally sensitive and respectful communication is essential when caring for women who have experienced FGM. This practice, although widely considered a human rights violation, is deeply rooted in culture and tradition in some areas of the world. Regarded as a rite of passage for young girls, FGM is thought to be performed to preserve purity and virginity prior to marriage, promote cleanliness, decrease promiscuity, or uphold cultural and religious traditions of a community. Families of young girls are often under great pressure to conform to local norms and risk being ostracized and/or having their daughters labeled as ineligible for marriage if FGM is not performed according to local traditions.

When discussing issues relating to sexual and reproductive health, providers must first determine the individual woman's feelings toward the procedure. The term "mutilation" is commonly used in Western culture to describe the level of alteration to the genitals, but some women may find this term offensive, especially if they view FGM as an important aspect of womanhood within their culture. Some women may prefer the term "cutting" when speaking of having the procedure done. Not all women will view FGM as abnormal and therefore may not be interested in genital reconstruction.

Follow-Up

Depending of the level of FGM, results of the exam, and patient complaints, some women may require a referral for surgical evaluation. Defibulation is the process of reconstructive surgery to open the scar that narrows the vaginal and urinary openings. Common reasons for requesting defibulation include a desire for pregnancy and vaginal delivery, relief from dyspareunia, and correction of urinary and menstrual difficulties. Referral for gynecologic evaluation under anesthesia may be necessary if the woman presents with symptoms that cannot be adequately diagnosed in a routine office visit. It is imperative to take into consideration patient preferences and exam findings when evaluating the need for referral.

FAST FACTS in a NUTSHELL

It is important to recognize that some women may not want corrective surgery, even in the presence of multiple adverse symptoms.

For further information related to specific pelvic exam challenges and potential resolutions, please see Appendix A.

PART

III

In-Office Diagnostic Testing

13

Performing In-Office Diagnostic Tests

INTRODUCTION

In-office testing for diagnosis and management of vulvovaginitis offers the opportunity to provide etiology-specific management at the time of the patient's visit. This contributes to rapid symptom relief for the patient and may prevent potential complications. "Out-of-office" commercial- or hospital-based diagnostic lab testing is increasingly popular. However, a significant disadvantage is that it requires several days to a week or longer (depending on the tests ordered) for results to return and subsequent etiology specific treatment to commence based on these results. This delay prolongs and, in some cases, can be associated with worsening symptoms, and patients may also be at risk for developing complications during this time. The "best practice" approach is to consider combining both in-office and commercial testing as indicated and most appropriate.

In this chapter you will learn how to:

1. Collect a vaginal sample for in-office testing for vaginal pH, amine testing, and vaginal microscopy.
2. Perform a vaginal pH test, using either a numerical or a new non-numerical test.
3. Conduct a potassium hydroxide (KOH), amine, "whiff" test.
4. Prepare, perform, and accurately interpret a vaginal microscopy, wet mount, or a "hanging drop" test.

VAGINAL SAMPLE COLLECTION

A vaginal sample used to for pH, amine/KOH, and vaginal microscopy testing is optimally collected from the posterior lateral vaginal wall. It is best to use a plastic Pap smear spatula; however, a cotton-tipped swab (two together is best) may also be used to collect the sample. A sample may also be collected from the edges of the speculum blades, being careful to avoid cervical mucus pooled in the lower speculum blade.

Vaginal pH Testing

Vaginal pH testing is used to screen for vaginitis. It is fairly sensitive but not as specific as blood, semen, cervical mucus, and certain vaginal medications (over-the-counter [OTC] and prescription) can alter results by falsely elevating the pH of the vagina. For example, semen, which is alkaline, can raise the vaginal pH for up to eight hours after intercourse.

The normal pH of the vagina is acidic, varying between 3.2 and 4.6. This normal pH correlates with a yellow color change in the pH paper after exposure to a sample of vaginal discharge. Several commercial pH testing systems use phen-aphthazine pH testing paper (Nitrazine, pHEM-Alert pH test [Femtek], Fem-V [Synova]), and these are all available to clinicians. These numerical pH tests are somewhat cumbersome for clinicians as they require a number of steps, including interpreting the color change accurately, which is not always easy.

Phenaphthazine Vaginal pH Testing Procedure
(Nitrazine, pHEM-Alert pH, Fem-V)

- Available in a multi-test roll, in container with pH color chart on cover
- Tear off 1-inch strip of pH paper (from roll)
- Place pH strip on paper towel next to pH color chart
  - Color chart on cover of pH paper container
- Apply vaginal sample to pH strip
- Match color to numerical pH on color chart
- Yellow = ~4.0, a normal vaginal pH
  - Limits differential to no vaginal infection, yeast, contact dermatitis, sexually transmitted infections (STIs), including HSV, unlikely to be bacterial vaginosis (BV), trichomoniasis, or atrophic vaginitis
- Green = ~5.0, possible BV and/or trichomoniasis and/or atrophic vaginitis
- Blue = ~6.0, possible trichomoniasis, atrophic vaginitis, semen, blood, or cervical mucus

The new non-numerical vaginal pH "VS-Sense" swab test, is now available in the United States. This swab test looks like a cotton-tipped applicator but with a yellow pH swab tip. The swab may be used to collect a lateral vaginal wall sample during the speculum exam, or may be inserted vaginally without the use of a speculum. Using the VS-Sense swab, a sample may also be taken from the edges of the speculum (after removal of the speculum), being careful to avoid cervical mucus pooled in the lower blades of the speculum.

When the swab is exposed to a sample of vaginal discharge, it turns color. If the vaginal pH is normal, the swab remains yellow. However, if the pH is abnormal, the swab turns blue, indicating possible bacterial vaginosis, trichomoniasis, or atrophic vaginitis. It may also be falsely elevated by semen or blood. The swab is buffered so it won't be falsely elevated by exposure to cervical mucus. This new "VS-Sense" swab test is quick, easy, and inexpensive (reimbursable and CLIA waived) and helps clinicians screen patients for vulvovaginitis. If the swab results are abnormal, it is recommended that further testing be done either in-office or sent to a lab.

There is only one OTC vaginal pH self-screening test for consumers. The "Vagisil" self-screening test is easy to use and tests whether a women's vaginal pH is normal or abnormal. If the pH is abnormal, patients are advised to seek medical attention to be evaluated for various types of vaginal infections and STIs.

Potassium Hydroxide (KOH), Amine, or "Whiff" Test

This test is used to screen for BV and involves mixing a sample of vaginal discharge with potassium hydroxide. The clinician immediately checks for a foul, fishy odor, indicating a positive test suggesting BV. This test is quite predictive for BV, being only inferior in accuracy to the presence of clue cells on vaginal microscopy.

KOH/Amine/Whiff Testing Procedure

- Mix a small amount of vaginal discharge with 10% to 20% KOH solution
  - Either on a glass slide or in a test tube, or drop onto a swab containing vaginal sample
- Note immediately, a positive result indicated by the presence of a foul, fishy odor
- A positive result represents one in four of Amsel's criteria for diagnosing BV

- The presence of three of four criteria is required for the diagnosis of BV per the 2010 Centers for Disease Control and Prevention STI Treatment Guidelines
  - These criteria include coaty white discharge, an elevated vaginal pH, a positive amine test, and clue cells on vaginal microscopy

═══════════════════════*FAST FACTS in a NUTSHELL*

Avoid adding KOH to saline mixed with vaginal sample, as this may result in a false negative test result due to the dilution of the vaginal mucus sample in the saline mixture.

Vaginal Microscopy Procedure, Wet Mount, Hanging Drop Test

Vaginal microscopy is still considered the "gold standard" test for diagnosing vulvovaginitis. Unfortunately, even when performed by a skilled clinician, the accuracy of this test is modest, at best, ranging from 60% to 80%. Requiring many steps, the sample must be obtained and prepared properly, then viewed correctly to achieve this accuracy.

Increasingly vaginal microscopy is being replaced by commercial testing systems that use polymerase chain reaction (PCR) technology that may include the following tests: Pap, HPV, and STI testing, in addition to testing for various types of vaginitis (BV, trichomoniasis, and candidiasis). These systems are referred to as "one collection, multiple detections" tests and offer quick, easy, accurate results usually within three to five days.

However, point-of-care testing with vaginal microscopy (and other in-office tests) offers the advantage of confirming the diagnosis at the time of the patient visit, facilitating prompt etiology-specific treatment, possibly resulting in more rapid relief of the patient's symptoms.

Vaginal Microscopy Procedure

- Using either a plastic spatula or two cotton-tipped applicators obtain a lateral vaginal wall sample

━━━━━━━━━━━━━━━━━━*FAST FACTS in a NUTSHELL*

A cotton-tipped applicator (or two for better sampling) may be used with or without the aid of a speculum exam to obtain a vaginal sample for microscopic analysis. Vaginal pH may be assessed in this manner also, using another swab to collect a sample.

- Wear gloves.
- Place one or two glass slides on a paper towel.
  - Apply 1 drop of saline to the left side of a glass slide.
  - Apply 1 drop of 10% to 20% KOH solution on the right side of the same glass slide; or two slides may be used, one for saline, one for KOH.
- Take the spatula containing sample or cotton tipped swabs and
  - Mix gently in saline until slightly opaque (dilute).
  - Mix sample in KOH, stirring until creamy white (concentrated).
- Immediately check for a foul, fishy odor indicating a positive amine result.
- Before viewing the smear on the microscope
  - Apply coverslips gently over saline sample and the KOH sample.
  - Avoid creating air bubbles by placing one side of coverslip on first.
- View saline smear under low power for adequacy of sample.
  - Six or more epithelial cells per low-power field (LPF)
  - And for general appearance, first impression (clue cells, WBCs, hyphae)

(continued)

(continued)

- View saline smear under high power to identify the following:
  - Yeast forms (hyphae and/or buds), clue cells, trichomonads
  - WBCs, RBCs, lactobacilli
  - Maturation of epithelial cells (superficial, large; intermediate, medium; or immature cells, small)
  - Numerous immature cells indicate either inflammation (trichomoniasis) and/or low estrogen levels (atrophy).
- To identify yeast, the KOH sample may be reviewed (if yeast is not noted on saline sample).
  - Look for hyphae (short, segmented), pseudophyphae (long, less segmented), and/or buds (spores).
  - Hyphae look like elongated circus balloons, with tapering along their lengths.
- To ensure modest accuracy, the vaginal smear is evaluated for two to three minutes.
  - Approximately 10 to 12 high-power fields (HPF) should be analyzed.
- Record your findings.
- Discard glass slides in a biohazard box.
- Maintain a clean microscope.
  - Wear gloves when cleaning the microscope.
  - The staging may be cleaned with an alcohol swab (where the glass slide is placed).
  - The low- and high-power magnifying objectives may be cleaned with a swab and saline, or lens paper/lens cleaner.

Common Pelvic Examination Problems and Interventions

Pelvic Examination Problem	Interventions
Extreme anxiety	Defer exam, palpate cervix before bimanual, step-by-step desensitization, relaxation techniques, deep breathing, anti-anxiety meds, counseling
Inability to insert speculum due to discomfort	Use Pederson or small speculum Use a swab to collect samples for Pap, STIs, wet mount; deep breathing Consider urine testing for STIs
Inability to insert speculum due to dryness	Palpate introital tissues or cervix before speculum insertion Apply scant lubricant to tip of speculum
Inability to insert speculum due to small and/or tight introitus	Palpate cervix; use small Pederson speculum or Dacron swab for STIs, wet mount; relaxation breathing
Inability to visualize cervix	Palpate cervix before speculum exam, move speculum side to side (shimmy), change angle slightly, instruct patient to bear down, try larger speculum, open wider
Vaginal walls impede visualizing cervix	Condom or glove over speculum (cut off tip) Use larger blade speculum like Graves or Clinton Graves, open wide Guttman or "Snowman" lateral vaginal wall retractor

(continued)

Pelvic Examination Problem	Interventions
Inability to view cervix because of extreme posterior position	Use large, extra-long speculum, open wide Like "Clinton Pederson" style Palpate cervix before Push down on suprapubic area Instruct patient to bear down Lift hips, spread thighs, knee stirrups
Speculum comes out unless clinician holds it	Seek an assistant to hold the speculum while you collect specimens, remove speculum, then prepare tests
Patient unable to tolerate speculum in situ secondary to anxiety and/or pain	Collect samples, remove speculum, then prepare tests Remember, samples are stable on sampling tools
History of sexual abuse and extreme phobia of pelvic exams–with or without vaginismus	Co-manage with a specialized counselor Use step-by-step desensitization program May not be able to complete a pelvic exam for several visits (may take months or years)

B

Vaginal Microscopy Flow Sheet

Date			
HPI			
LMP, last coitus			
Vulva, vagina, cervix			
Vaginal mucus			
Cervical mucus			
pH (4.0–7.5) <4.7 = normal			
Amine test (KOH)			
Wet mount (saline)			
Low power (quality)			
High power (detail)			
LB (0–3+)			
Bacteria (0–3+)			
WBCs (0–3+)			
Other			
Wet mount (KOH)			
Low power			
High power			
Assessment			
Plan			

C

Vaginal Microscopy: Flow Sheet Instructions

Date	
CC, HPI	Brief history of symptoms including self-care, meds
LMP, last coitus	Last menstrual period, last coitus, dyspareunia
Vulva, vagina, cervix	Erythema, lesions, tenderness
Vaginal mucus	Amount and characteristics
Cervical mucus	Color, quality, amount
pH (4.0–7.5) (<4.7 = normal)	Use 1 inch strip of Nitrazine or ColorpHast paper dip pH paper into vaginal mucus collected on spatula or swab
Amine test (10% KOH)	Using spatula with sample, stir x10 into 20% KOH on glass slide (use 2 slides, 1 for KOH, 1 for saline); check fishy, foul odor
Wet mount (saline) (dilute w/scattered ECs)	Using wooden spatula containing sample, stir x3 into saline solution on glass slide
Low power (quality) x10 magnification	General appearance and quality of sample, for example, proper concentration, too diluted, too concentrated
High power (detail) x40 magnification	Identify organisms and morphology
LB= lactobacilli (0–3+); appear as rods	1+ = few, 2 = dominant, 3+ = false clue cells

(continued)

Bacteria=anaerobes (0–3+) appear as tiny cocci	1+ = few per HPF, 2+ = dominant background per HPF 3+ = clue cells
WBC's (0–3+) size of nucleus of an EC	1+ = 1:1 ratio to EC's, 2+ = 5:1, 3+ = 10:1 or greater
Other, including epithelial cells (ECs)	ECs (true clue cells, false clue cells, superficial, parabasal, basal) yeast, trich, mobiluncus, sperm, RBCs, medications, artifact
Wet mount (KOH; very concentrated)	ECs look like round, hollow, balloons called ghost cells
Low power	Hyphael forms (cobwebs) visible but not buds
High power	Hyphae = look like elongated circus balloons Buds = spherical glass beads, slightly different size, shapes
Assessment	Specify including rule outs, list most likely to least likely
Plan	Dx tests including yeast cultures, meds, education, follow-up

D

Vulvar Care Guidelines
for Patient Education

- For vulvar itching
  - <u>Hydrocortisone 1% **ointment**</u> over-the-counter
    - Apply twice a day as needed (no limit on how long you can use)
  - Clobetasol or halobetasol 0.05% ointment (if prescribed)
    - Apply daily for 2 weeks, then every other day for 2–4 weeks, then twice weekly as needed
  - Apply <u>Vaseline,</u> "Crisco," or pure mineral oil daily or more often
  - Increase use as you taper the Clobetasol or Hydrocortisone
- Vulvar care basics: "Less is more"—DO NOT SCRUB
  - Wash with warm water
  - AVOID washing with SOAP
  - May use <u>mineral oil</u> as a soap substitute (pure unscented—NOT baby oil)
  - Avoid shaving: especially near the vagina—trimming hair is okay
- Wear all cotton underwear OR synthetic undies with cotton crotch insert
  - <u>Avoid thong underwear:</u> may cause bacteria to move from "back to front"
  - Wash in HOT water, double rinse
  - Use ½ the soap recommended

- Avoid intercourse during treatment AND while you are having symptoms
  - <u>Avoid sex if painful</u>
  - Use condoms when possible
- Wipe from "front to back"
- Sex
  - Wash hands and partner's hands/penis before sex
  - Use <u>water-based lubricants such as KY products</u>
    - <u>Unscented, unflavored,</u> "Silke," "Intrigue," "Slippery Stuff"
  - Use condoms; especially with anal intercourse
    - Use a new condom for vaginal intercourse
  - Wash sex toys
  - Try to maintain a similar pattern of sexual activity over time
- Avoid douching; the vagina is self-cleaning
- Vitamin D_3: Take 1,000–2,000 IU daily (calcium 1,000 mg daily)
- Reduce your stress
- Increase sleep
- Sleep without underwear; wear loose clothing during day, especially avoid tight jeans
- Return when recommended and if symptoms persist or recur

References

Abdulcadir, J., Margairaz, C., Boulvain, M., & Irion, O. (2011). Care of women with female genital mutilation/cutting. *Swiss Medical Weekly, 140*, 1–8.

ACOG Committee on Practice Bulletins—Gynecology. (2009). ACOG Practice Bulletin No. 109: Cervical cytology screening. *Obstetrics and Gynecology, 114*, 1409–1420.

Bates, C. K., Carroll, N., & Potter, J. (2010). The challenging pelvic examination. *The Journal of General Internal Medicine, 26*(6), 651–657.

Braddy, C. M., & Files, J. A. (2007). Female genital mutilation: Cultural awareness and clinical considerations. *Journal of Midwifery and Women's Health, 52*, 158–163.

Brown, K. M., & Muscari, M. E. (2010). *Quick reference to adult and older adult forensics: A guide for nurses and other health care professionals* (p. 170). New York, NY: Springer Publishing Company.

Centers for Disease Control and Prevention. (2010). Sexually transmitted diseases guidelines, 2010. *Morbidity and Mortality Weekly Report, 59*(RR-12), 1–114.

Carcio, H. A., & Secor, M. C. (2010). *Advanced health assessment of women: Clinical skills and procedures* (2nd ed.). New York, NY: Springer Publishing Company.

Cash, J. C., & Glass, C.A. (2010). *Family practice guidelines* (2nd ed.). New York, NY: Springer Publishing Company.

Centers for Disease Control and Prevention. (2010). U.S. medical eligibility criteria for contraceptive use: Adapted from the World Health Organization medical eligibility criteria for contraceptive use (4th ed.). *Morbidity and Mortality Weekly Report, 59* (RR-4).

Chelmow, D., Waxman, A., Cain, J. M., & Lawrence, H. C., III. (2012). The evolution of cervical screening and the specialty of obstetrics and gynecology [Abstract]. *Obstetrics and Gynecology, 119,* 695–699.

Fogel, C. I., & Woods, N. F. (2008). *Woman's health care in advanced practice nursing.* New York, NY: Springer Publishing Company.

Giadino, A. P., Datner, E. M., & Asher, J. B. (2003). *Sexual assault victimization: Across the lifespan.* St. Louis, MO: JW Medical.

Hamoudi, A., & Shier, M. (2010). Late complications of childhood female genital mutilation. *Journal of Obstetrics and Gynaecology Canada, 32,* 587–589.

Harmanli, O., & Jones, K. A. (2010). Using lubricant for speculum insertion. *Obstetrics and Gynecology, 116,* 415–417.

Hawkins, J. W., Roberto-Nichols, D. M., & Stanley-Haney, J. L. (2011). *Guidelines for nurse practitioners in gynecologic settings* (10th ed.). New York, NY: Springer Publishing Company.

Jarvis, C. (2008). *Physical examination and health assessment* (5th ed.). St. Louis, MO: Saunders.

Logan, T. K., Walker, R., & Hunt, G. (2009). Understanding human trafficking in the United States. *Trauma, Violence, and Abuse, 10*(3), 3–30. doi: 10.1177/15249=838008327262

McClain, N. M., & Garrity, S. E. (2011). Sex trafficking and the exploitation of adolescents. *Journal of Obstetrics, Gynecologic, and Neonatal Nursing, 40,* 243–252. doi: 10.1111/j.1552-6909 .2011.01221.x

Momoh, C. (2010). Female genital mutilation. *Trends in Urology, Gynaecology & Sexual Health, 15,* 11–14.

Moyer, V. A. (2012). On behalf of the US Preventive Services Task Force. Screening for cervical cancer: US Preventive Services Task Force recommendation statement. *Annals of Internal Medicine* [Epub ahead of print] http://www.annals.org/content/early/2012/03/14/ 0003-4819-156-12-201206190-00424.full?sid=46a1b5af-88a2- 4d47-9c5e-76cb8ba67206

Nelson, A., & Rubin, M. (2011). Anal dysplasia. *Female Patient, 36,* 1–5.

Rhoads, J. (2006). *Advanced health assessment and diagnostic reasoning.* Philadelphia, PA: Lippincott Williams & Wilkins.

Richman, S. M., & Drickamer, M. A. (2007). Gynecologic care of elderly women. *Journal of the American Medical Directors Association, 8*(4), 219–223.

Saslow, D., et al. (2012). American Cancer Society, American Society for Colposcopy and Cervical Pathology, and American Society for Clinical Pathology screening guidelines for the prevention and early detection of cervical cancer. *American Journal of Clinical Pathology, 137*, 516.

Secor, M. (1998). The gynecologic exam. In H. Carcio (Ed.), *Infertility for the primary care provider.* Philadelphia, PA: Lippincott-Raven.

Sommers, M. (2007). Defining patterns of genital injury from sexual assault: A review. *Trauma, Violence, & Abuse, 8*(3), 270–280.

Tanner, J. M. (1962). *Growth at adolescence.* Oxford, England: Blackwell Scientific.

Tjaden, P., & Thoennes, N. (2000). *Full report of the prevalence, incidence, and consequences of violence against women: Findings from the National Violence Against Women survey* (NCJ183781). Washington, DC: National Institute of Justice, Office of Justice Programs, U.S. Department of Justice. Retrieved from www.ncjrs.gov/peffiles 1/nij/183781.pdf

U.S. Cancer Statistics Working Group. (2010). *United States Cancer Statistics: 1999–2007 Incidence and Mortality Web-Based Report.* Atlanta, GA: Department of Health and Human Services, Centers for Disease Control and Prevention, and National Cancer Institute. Retrieved from http://www.cdc.gov/uscs

U.S. Department of Health and Human Services. (2009). *Resources: Common health issues seen in victims of human trafficking. Look Beneath the Surface: Restore and Rescue.* Retrieved from www.acf.hhs.gov/trafficking/index.html

U.S. Department of State. (2006). *Trafficking in persons report.* Washington, DC: Author. Retrieved from www.state.gov/g/tip/rls/tiprpt/2006/

Wee, C. C., McCartney, E. P., Davis, R. B., & Phillips, R. S. (2000). Screening for cervical and breast cancer: Is obesity an unrecognized barrier to preventive care? *Annals of Internal Medicine, 132*, 697–704.

Weitlauf, J. C., Finney, J. W., Ruzek, J., Lee, T. T., Thrailkill, A., Jones, S., & Frayne, S. M. (2008). Distress and pain during pelvic examinations: Effect of sexual violence. *Obstetrics & Gynecology, 112*, 1343–1350.

World Health Organization. (2008). *Eliminating female genital mutilation: An interagency statement.* Geneva, Switzerland: Author.

Wright, T. C., Jr., et al. (2007). 2006 ASCCP-Sponsored Consensus Conference. 2006 consensus guidelines for the management of women with abnormal cervical screening tests [Abstract]. *Journal of Lower Genital Tract Disease, 11,* 201–222.

RESOURCES

Cervical cancer screening guidelines

www.uspreventiveservicestaskforce.org/uspstf11/cervcancer/cervcancerupd.htm

www.asccp.org

www.acog.org

Contraceptive guidelines

2010 CDC Contraceptive Medical Eligibility Criteria

www.cdc/contraceptivemedicaleligibilitycriteria

www.cdc.gov/mmwr/preview/mmwrhtml/mm6026a3.htm?s_cid=mm6026a3_w

Menopause information

North American Menopause Association

www.nams.org

Sexually transmitted infections

2010 CDC STD Treatment Guidelines

www.cdc.gov/std/treatment/2010/default.htm

Abbreviations

ASC-H	suspect high grade lesion
ASC-US	atypical squamous cells of unclear significance
AVB	abnormal vaginal bleeding
BMD	bone mineral density
BMI	body mass index
BV	bacterial vaginosis
CA125	cancer antigen 125
CAD	coronary artery disease
CBC	complete blood count
CHF	congestive heart failure
CIN	cervical intraepithelial neoplasia
CMT	cervical motion tenderness
CVA	cerebral vascular accidents
CVA	costovertebral angle
CVAT	costovertebral angle tenderness
DES	diethylstilbestrol
DUB	dysfunctional uterine bleeding
EC	epithelial cell
EMR	electronic medical record
E-stim	electrical stimulation
FGM	female genital mutilation (also called female circumcision or female cutting)
FLP	fasting lipid profile
FSH	follicle-stimulating hormone
GI	gastrointestinal
HIPAA	Health Insurance Portability and Accountability Act of 1996
HIV	human immunodeficiency virus

HPF	high-power field
HPV	human papillomavirus
HRA	high resolution anoscopy
HR-HPV	high-risk human papillomavirus
HSIL	high grade squamous intraepithelial lesion
IGG	immune globulin G
KOH	potassium hydroxide
LH	luteinizing hormone
LMP	last menstrual period
LP	lichen planus
LPF	low-power field
LS	lichen sclerosis
LSC	lichen simplex chronicus
LSIL	low grade squamous intraepithelial lesion
MI	myocardial infarction
MDL	Medical Diagnostic Laboratories
MRSA	methicillin-resistant *Staphylococcus aureus*
MSM	men who have sex with men
NAAT	nucleic acid amplification testing
NSSC	normal size, shape, contour
NVAWS	National Violence Against Women Survey
OAB	overactive bladder
OTC	over-the-counter
Pap	Papanicolaou
PC	pubococcygeal
PCOS	polycystic ovarian syndrome
PCR	polymerase chain reaction
PID	pelvic inflammatory disease
POS	polycystic ovarian syndrome
PUPP	pruritic urticarial papules of pregnancy
RBC	red blood cell count
ROS	review of systems
RPR	rapid plasma reagin (syphilis test)
STI	sexually transmitted infection
TSH	thyroid-stimulating hormone
UTI	urinary tract infection
VIN	vulvar intraepithelial neoplasia
VMS	vasomotor symptoms
WBC	white blood cell
WHO	World Health Organization

Index

CPSIA information can be obtained
at www.ICGtesting.com
Printed in the USA
LVHW081001180119
604400LV00014B/223/P

9 780826 107800